THE MOLECULES WITHIN US

Our Body in Health and Disease

THE MOLECULES WITHIN US

Our Body in Health and Disease

Dr. Charles A. Pasternak

PLENUM TRADE • NEW YORK AND LONDON

Library of Congress Cataloging-in-Publication Data

Pasternak, Charles A. (Charles Alexander)
    The molecules within us : our body in health and disease / Charles
A. Pasternak.
       p.   cm.
    Includes bibliographical references and index.
    ISBN 0-306-45987-6
    1. Biochemistry. 2. Molecular biology. 3. Medicine. 4. Human
physiology.   I. Title.
    [DNLM: 1. Physiology. 2. Biochemistry. 3. Molecular Biology.
QT 104P291m 1998]
QP514.2.P374   1998
610--dc21
DNLM/DLC
for Library of Congress   98-26173
                                                                  CIP

ISBN 0-306-45987-6

© 1998 Charles A. Pasternak
Plenum Press is a Division of Plenum Publishing Corporation
233 Spring Street, New York, N.Y. 10013

http://www.plenum.com

10 9 8 7 6 5 4 3 2 1

To Helen and Bill Ramsay
for their hospitality during the writing of this book
and for constant support

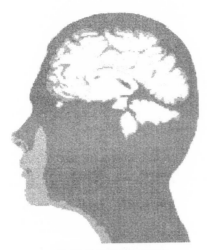

CONTENTS

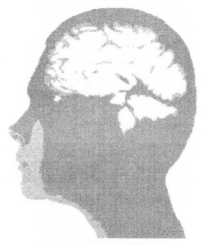

FOREWORD

The average citizen who is concerned about health matters is likely to view the output of present day medical researchers with an uncomfortable ambivalence, pleased to learn that tax dollars and other public support are being put to productive uses, but perplexed by an inability to understand exactly what has been achieved.

Part of the problem is certainly a matter of communication. Scientists make discoveries using the tools of chemistry, physics, and biology, and their findings are best revealed to others, using the most appropriate technical terms. To the experienced practitioner who deals with them on a daily basis, these terms are effective ways to transmit complex ideas simply and faithfully. But to the uninitiated, these terms are as inaccessible as a foreign language. To suggest, for example, that a gene has been discovered that causes cell cycle arrest, through a frameshift mutation, would be readily understood by a modern cancer researcher, but completely unintelligible to someone not familiar with the terms gene, cell cycle arrest, and frameshift mutation.

The most dramatic advances in medicine are often described by journalists and others, but, because so much of the rich technical detail is omitted, such accounts often lack the excitement of discovery. Those who do try to provide some appreciation of the science involved are usually forced to choose between the vernacular of the specialist, which is often opaque to the general reader, or more user-friendly but less precise everyday metaphors.

Scientists who study living organisms have found that complex biological systems can be more readily understood if the individual building blocks that make up each cell and tissue are isolated and analyzed at the molecular level. Biologists, working at the level of molecules, refer to themselves as molecular biologists. Indeed, a whole new field of molecular medicine has evolved within the past decade.

Members of the public can experience the afterglow of these exciting new developments, but only if they acquire a working understanding of what biological molecules actually are. This volume, an account of what molecules are and how they both function and misfunction, is a welcome step in this direction. People long absent from the classroom will finally learn exactly what DNA is and how it influences every aspect of the living body, from nose shape to memory. They will learn how DNA can go "bad," often due to avoidable environmental influences, and result in cancer, heart disease, or degeneration of the nervous system.

Armed with these new insights the public will be better able to appreciate why the United States government is investing billions of dollars in the Human Genome Project. And when it is completed, those who take the trouble to learn what molecules are and how they work will be able to decide for themselves what genetics may mean for their health and welfare in the future.

Wading through this insightful book will be well worth the effort.

Vincent T. Marchesi
Director
Boyer Center for Molecular Medicine
Yale University

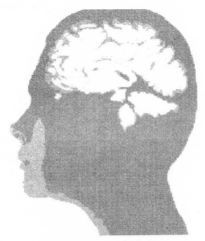

FOREWORD

B iomedical knowledge has advanced more rapidly in the past 50 years than in the preceding 5000 years, and we are at last coming to know in some detail how our body works, and what we can do about it if it begins to fail. This position has been reached because we now understand in molecular terms—terms of molecules like glucose and cholesterol, DNA and proteins—exactly how the food that we eat is turned into the cells that make up our bodies, how the energy inherent in the oxidation of food drives our muscles and heart, how organs like kidney, liver, and brain and the nervous system all work in a coordinated manner. We can also treat disease in a rational manner, with drugs tailor-made to restore faulty organs to normal function, with antibiotics to kill infectious bacteria, and with vaccines to stop bacteria, viruses, and other microbes, from ever infecting us in the first place, and—still around the corner—with therapies that restore faulty genes to their full potential.

Much of this knowledge has been locked up in scientific and medical publications to which the average person has no access. Now, for the first time, Charles Pasternak has explained the detailed workings of our bodies in health and disease with such clarity that it has opened up an understanding of the molecular basis of life to everyone. And it is important for everyone to understand these matters, for important decisions regarding embryonic technologies, gene therapy, and the knowledge of a person's makeup, need to be made not by scientists and medical doctors, but by the public at large. It is fortunate that Charles Pasternak's lucid exposition of *The Molecules Within Us* has appeared at such a timely moment. I recommend everyone with an interest in how their bodies work, and what they can do about it, to read this narrative: You will certainly be fascinated by it.

(Sir) John Vane
Nobel Laureate
Honorary President
The William Harvey Research Institute
London

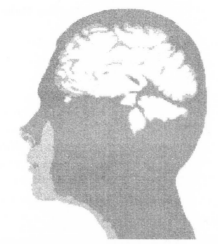

ACKNOWLEDGMENTS

I am grateful to many friends and colleagues for fruitful discussion of some of the issues raised in this book and for supplying—sometimes prior to publication—certain information. If the interpretations I have suggested are faulty, the blame is entirely mine. These kind people include Richard Asser, Lindsay Bashford, Robert Balasz, Richard Bethell, Nick Birch, Gerard Bodeker, Paul Calabresi, Jack Cooper, John Ellis, Mark Fisher, Lynn Fitzgerald, Mickey Gaitonde, Donald Gillies, Steve Goodbourn, Alan Johnstone, Dennis Lucas, Max Perutz, Richard Peto, Robert Plomin, Paul Richardson, John Skehel, Jamshed Tata, Richard Vile, and Herbert Wiener. To John Axford, Angus Dalgleish, John Griffiths, and Andrew Steptoe I owe an especial debt of gratitude for reading entire chapters or the whole typescript.

The bibliography at the end of the book suggests some further reading material on certain topics. It is not a comprehensive list of the sources I have consulted. I should therefore like to acknowledge the fact that many snippets of information came from the newspapers of the day, in particular from *The Times* and *Sunday Times*, published in the United Kingdom.

The illustrations that accompany this book were assembled with the help of Kristina Fallenius of the Nobel Foundation in Stockholm, who lent me many photographs of Nobel Laureates; of William Shubach of the Wellcome Institute for the History of Medicine in London; and of others who are acknowledged in the respective figure legends. I am particularly grateful to Duncan Larkin for providing new drawings and to Glenn Alder for help in assembling all the illustrations; they are both at St George's Medical School in London.

To my nephew Nick Ramsay I am grateful for lending me a lap-top computer on which much of this book was written. To my editor Linda Greenspan Regan at Plenum I owe a particular debt for her words of advice on the entire typescript. And without her colleagues at Plenum—especially Robert Maged, this work would never have found its way into print.

I could not have written this book without the support of two other people. One is Mike Clemens, Chairman of Biochemistry at St. George's Medical School, who graciously allowed me to retain my office after I had handed over the reins of power to him. The other is Stefanina Pelc, my secretary and personal assistant, without whom I am a lost soul in the idiosyncratic ways of e-mail and the Internet, and who always managed to rescue me when computers and printers conspired against me. It is she, also, who efficiently kept the other activities of my office in play while I was was frolicking with The Molecules Within Us.

Cortijo Grande, Almeria, Spain, and London, England, UK

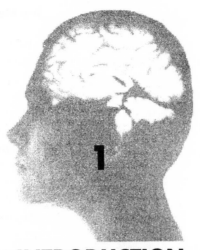

INTRODUCTION

Some years ago, during a scientific discussion at the weekend residence of former British Prime Minister Margaret Thatcher, one of her senior Cabinet members asked the question: "These molecules you talk about: what exactly are they? If I put some into a box, will they still be there in 10 days—or 10 years—time?" That question revealed an astonishing ignorance of elementary science, namely, that all matter is made up of molecules—whether it is the wood of the box or the air inside it—and that molecules remain intact unless they are changed to other molecules by chemical reactions. Although the politician concerned was a well-educated man—the Fellow of an Oxford College, no less—he was obviously ignorant of scientific principles taught to every schoolchild. He had also forgotten that Democritus, a philosopher whose work must have been known to him, had postulated the molecular nature of matter and had coined the word *atom* some 2400 years ago, though it took 2300 more years to prove it.

The point of this anecdote is not to question the wisdom of Margaret Thatcher's political appointment, but to conclude that there are many people who are confused these days by talk of "molecular complexity," "molecular modeling," "designer molecules," and so forth. Since every part of our body is made up of molecules, and since it is the chemical reactions between them that underlie our ailments as well as our well-being, it would seem worthwhile to summarize this for the lay reader, and perhaps student also. For it is knowledge of the interplay of molecules within us that allows scientists to make better drugs, and clinicians to diagnose and to treat us more effectively; but most of all, that knowledge allows every one of us to control our own health through an appropriate choice of diet, through avoidance of infectious disease, and through an awareness of the nature of stress.

For thousands of years we have been trying to understand how our bodies work. The Sumerians who lived in Babylon in Mesopotamia (now Iraq) 5000 years ago began to study the human body scientifically, and by 1600 B.C. the ancient Egyptians, who acquired much of their knowledge from this cradle of civilization, had a surprisingly good knowledge of anatomy, pharmacy, and pathology. The Greeks of 2500 years ago (a century before Democritus) recognized four elements that dominate life: earth (cold and dry), fire (hot and dry), water (cold and wet), and air (hot and wet). The Chinese, who had been practicing acupuncture already for 2500 years prior to this time, took a somewhat similar view. Five elements—water, fire, wood, metal, and earth—were recognized, but the principles of yin and yang, which have persisted up to the present day in traditional Chinese medicine, rather overshadowed them. Yin and yang represent opposite characteristics: Yin is negative, dark, female, wet, water, cold, night, moon, earth, and underactive (these are just examples; the concept of opposites is limitless), whereas yang is positive, light, male, dry, fire, hot, day, sun, heaven, and overactive. Life and our body is a delicate mixture of yin and yang. This concept has a reality in molecular terms, as will be appreciated in our discussion of the immune system and of stress.

Originally all medicine was tied up with magic, and the shaman or medicine man has persisted up to the present day in primitive—and not so primitive—societies. By around 400 B.C., the Greek philosopher Hippocrates of Cos was already challenging the view that disease results from supernatural causes and attributed it to the diet instead—another concept that has survived, in part, to the present day. Aristotle accepted the radical views of Hippocrates: "a great physician," though he could not refrain from adding "but a man of short stature." Within the next 200 years the followers of Hippocrates, many working in the Egyptian city of Alexandria, were identifying organs like heart, nerves, and brain, and one Erasistratus from Ceos went so far as to postulate that the heart is the motor for the circulation. In Rome the physician Galen of Pergamum had come to realize that the arteries contained not just air, but also blood. This was probably the first inkling of the importance of blood as a carrier for the oxygen that we inhale into our lungs. Galen more or less assumed the mantle of Hippocrates and became the most influential doctor of his day. Partly this was achieved by the force with which he expressed his authoritarian views: Do we not recognize this trait in many politicians—and scientists—of our day, who succeed where others fail simply because they express their views with such apparent certainty? But it has to be said that Galen was probably the first to open up the field of physiology through direct experimentation. Medicine was now definitely on the move. By the time that the Sung dynasty of China was at its height— just before being overrun by Genghis Khan and the Mongols in the twelfth century—dentistry, laryngology, obstetrics, and ophthalmology were being practiced alongside acupuncture in that most innovative of countries.

The Arab philosophers and scientists of the ninth century onwards accepted much of Greek medicine and the teachings of Galen. It was the Arabs who kept medicine, as well as other knowledge and the arts, alive throughout the centuries that marked the Dark Ages in Europe. The followers of Mohammed were not without contributions themselves. Rhazes, a Persian born in 850, was the first to distinguish measles from smallpox; although this was a scientific achievement of note, its usefulness was limited, as sufferers from either disease had to wait another 800 years for treatment. Another Persian, Avicenna (or Ibn Sinā, born in 980), was probably the first to apply what is today called psychotherapy. He cured an insane prince—who thought he was a cow and wanted to be slaughtered—by suggesting that he was too thin and needed fattening up first. The prince agreed, and as he became stronger his delusion left him. Avicenna also wrote a standard text—the *Canon of Medicine*—that remained in use in the medical schools of Europe until well into the seventeenth century. The Mayans of Central America, who had come to their peak in terms of astronomy, mathematics, and architecture by 900 A.D., did not practice much medicine. What they did practice, in contrast, was human sacrifice.

By the seventeenth century, then, knowledge of the various organs of the body—heart, liver, lungs, intestines—was pretty well established. What was lacking was insight into how they actually *worked*. The heart had come to be recognized as playing a central role: If it beats, one is alive; if it stops, one is dead. In 1628 William Harvey (Figure 1), an Englishman who had been trained in the Italian town of Padua, showed that the beating of the heart pushes blood around the body and that all of the blood pushed

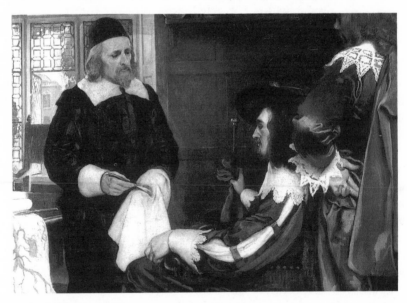

1. William Harvey. In this picture by Ernest Board, Harvey is demonstrating the circulation of the blood to King Charles I. Courtesy of The Wellcome Institute Library, London.

out of the heart eventually returns to it; in short, that we have a closed circulation of blood, in the way that a closed circulation of hot water underlies the working of a central heating system. Just as a pump is required to drive water through a boiler hooked up to a series of radiators, so the heart is required to drive blood through the lungs—where it picks up oxygen—and then to drive oxygenated blood through the rest of the body. Interestingly, Harvey used not mammals like mice or dogs for this work, but snakes. He reasoned, correctly, that all animals that contain blood and have a beating heart probably operate in the same way; by working with a cold-blooded animal like a snake, he was able to keep the heart going much longer after he had exposed it at the temperature of the room in which he was working, than would have been the case with a warm-blooded animal, which would have required a special room heated to 37°C to keep it alive. (Harvey knew about animals: In his writings, he refers to observations on bees, carp, caterpillars, crayfish, dogs, dolphin, eel, flies, frogs, goose, hen, hornet, horse, lizard, lobster, mice, mussels, ox, oyster, partridge, pig, pigeons, seals, sheep, shrimp, slug, snail, snake, swan, toad, tortoise, wasp, whale, and woodcock.) The actual experiment he performed was simple enough; if he tied off the vessels on one side of the heart (now known as the pulmonary arteries), the heart became swollen; if he tied off the vessels on the other side (now known as the systemic veins), it shrank: Ergo, blood flows in a circle (hence the word circulation), with the heart providing the necessary driving force.

The following three centuries saw the basic principles of anatomy (or structure) and physiology (or function) of the rest of the human body being refined and established. At the same time two advances revolutionized medicine. The first was the recognition—long suspected—that illnesses like the plague are spread by contact with diseased humans or animals. The existence of microbes had been established by the Dutch amateur scientist Antonie van Leeuwenhoek, 1632–1723 (Figure 2), who built the first microscope powerful enough to observe these organisms—animalcules—swimming in a glass of water. To Leeuwenhoek's surprise, he saw similar organisms in a sample of his own saliva (he was also the first to observe spermatozoa under the microscope).

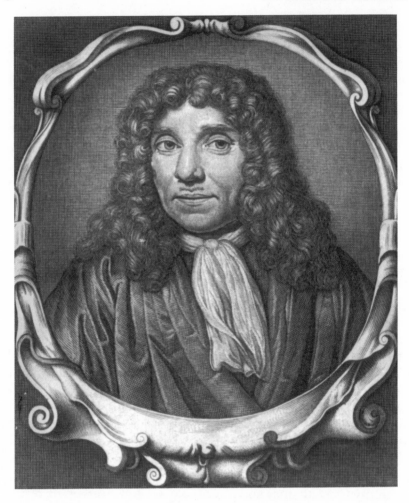

2. Antonie van Leeuwenhoek. Line engraving by A. de Blois after J. Verkolje.
Courtesy of The Wellcome Institute Library, London.

It took another 200 years for men like Robert Koch in Germany
(Figure 3) and Louis Pasteur in France (Figure 4) to show con-
vincingly that infectious microbes are indeed the causes of diseases such as anthrax, cholera, and tuberculosis, and to develop
vaccines that protect against the respective illnesses. (A vaccine
is, as we shall see in a later chapter, a preparation derived from

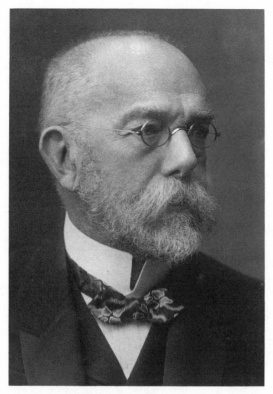

3. Robert Koch. Nobel laureate, 1905. Copyright: The Nobel Foundation, Stockholm.

an infectious microbe. When injected into the body it provides immunity against that very microbe.)

The second advance was the development of anesthetics to enable surgeons—and dentists—to operate without causing pain. It was the discovery of simple gaseous molecules such as nitrous oxide, chloroform, and ether during the late nineteenth and early twentieth centuries that led to their use, once the chemists who had synthesized the molecules had experienced their soporific value by inhaling them. Both advances—the realization that microbes are present on our skin as well as on the surgeon's knife or dentist's pliers, and that sterility is of prime importance during the removal of a limb, tumor, or tooth, cou-

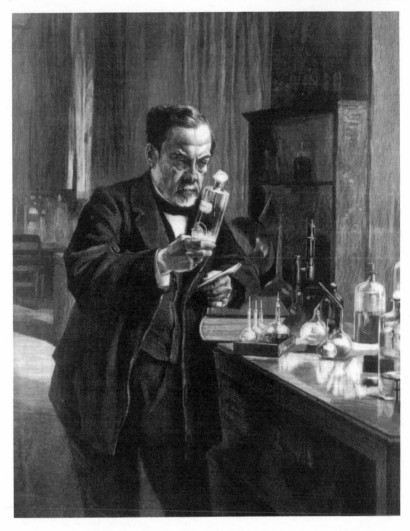

4. Louis Pasteur. Engraving of Pasteur in his laboratory, by Baude after Edelfelt. Courtesy of The Wellcome Institute Library, London.

pled with the use of anesthetics to ease the pain—have transformed surgeons and dentists from being barbers with a side interest in medicine, to being among the most respected (and highly paid) members of the medical profession.

The reason why it was not until the present century that the molecular nature underlying form and function started to be revealed is that analysis of the reactions that take place in the tissues of the body requires that the cells that make up those tissues be alive, and cutting out organs of breathing humans has never been part of our scientific endeavor. During the nineteenth century, however, it became clear that animals and humans are closely related and this has led to the use of animal tissues—rapidly removed the minute the animal is killed—for studying metabolic processes: processes such as the oxidation of foodstuffs, using the energy derived from the oxidation of food to fuel the contraction of muscles and the pumping of ions like Na^+ (sodium), K^+ (potassium), and Ca^{2+} (calcium) across cell membranes, and the synthesis of nucleic acids, proteins, carbohydrates, and fats. Answers now began to emerge to questions like *why* do muscle, nerve, and bone have different properties, and *how* does the heart pump blood or the intestines absorb food and water? To return to the analogy of the central heating system, *why* do radiators and the pipes that connect them have different properties in terms of heat radiation and heat conservation, and *how* is the water inside the boiler heated up and *how* does a circulating pump actually work? Of course explaining anatomy and physiology, or engineering materials and machines, in molecular terms is merely going to one further level of complexity. Why not go to the next level and try to explain everything not in terms of molecules—i.e., of chemistry—but in terms of neutrons, protons, and electrons—i.e., in terms of subatomic physics? The answer is that that would not be very useful with respect to the human body. For it is at the molecular level, the level of carbohydrate, cholesterol, and protein, that we can control our diet and it is at the molecular level, of aspirin, Prozac, or penicillin, that we can ameliorate pain, depression, or a bacterial infection. In the same way it is metallurgy—the chemistry of metals—and not subatomic physics that is of practical use to engineers today.

There is another reason why it took more than 300 years from the time of William Harvey to describe the workings of the heart in terms of molecules, i.e., in terms of proteins like myosin and actin, of calcium, and of ATP (adenosine triphosphate: the molecular fuel for all energy-requiring reactions). The answer is that scientific discovery and insight progress only when the necessary techniques are at hand. As many Nobel prizes, for example, have been won for establishing a new methodology, as for exploiting existing techniques to elucidate previously obscure processes like energy metabolism or nerve conduction. And chemistry—the study of matter and its interactions at the level of molecules—did not begin until the late eighteenth and early nineteenth centuries. It was only in the 1950s that methods were developed to study molecules in the relatively low numbers present in animal cells. The impetus for this advance owes its origin to two factors. First was the realization that many metabolic reactions are the same in microbes as in animals and man; the ease of growing and studying nonpathogenic, i.e., non-disease-causing, bacteria has made *Escherichia coli*—together with rat liver—the subjects of choice for biochemists. The second factor was World War II (1939–1945). For it was the development of the atomic bomb during that war that led to the synthesis and use of radioactive compounds: radioactively "tagged" molecules like glucose and amino acids that can be detected in extremely low amounts. This is a prerequisite for mapping the molecular changes that take place in cells. Thus, the development of the greatest weapon of mass destruction known to man led—in an entirely unpredictable way—to deeper knowledge of how our body works and hence of ways to combat disease in a rational, and thus more effective, manner.

This book is an attempt to explain to the general reader what kinds of molecules underlie our bodily functions and how these molecules interact in health and disease. I begin with a brief description of the molecules of living matter and then discuss how they participate in nutrition and metabolism; in order to do that the reader will be reminded of the main organs that make up the human body—heart, liver, kidney, muscle, and brain—and the molecular changes that underlie the way they work. Next I consider the nature–versus–nurture debate: To what extent is our body—whether we are fat or thin, intelligent or stupid—dependent on the genes we inherit from our parents, and to what extent is it dependent on the food we eat and other environmental factors? And more important, are the illnesses from which we suffer, like heart disease or cancer, a consequence of our genes or of the environment in which we live? Some diseases, to be sure, are environmental: We have only to move into a tropical region to be aware of that, and the coughs and colds that beset us in winter are not related to our genetic makeup either. But why is it that some of us survive infections better than others and how are any of us able to recover from an infectious episode at all? The answers to these questions have come from the realization that there exists within us a system—known as the immune system— that is able to fight infections and eventually rid the body of the offending microbe. It is because of subtle differences in people's immune systems that one person may succumb to an infection that leaves another person unaffected.

Next I turn to one of the most talked about illnesses of our age, namely, stress. What exactly is stress, how does it affect our bodies, and what can we do about it? This brings us to a general discussion of how to treat disease. What do we know of the molecular changes underlying alternative treatments like acupuncture or herbal medicines and do they have a place in a world of heart transplants, designer vaccines, and novel antidepressant drugs? And now on to one of the least understood areas of the body, the brain. What is the molecular basis of pain and pleasure, of learning and memory, of grief and joy? What is the likelihood that we shall find a cure for schizophrenia, multiple sclerosis, or Alzheimer's disease? Finally, as every reader sadly knows (unless he believes in reincarnation), we are on this earth for a very limited period of time. Unlike the bristlecone trees of southern California that live for over 1000 years, our life span is at best some 100 years. What are the causes of our eventual demise, and can we hold them at bay with novel drugs and therapies?

These, then, are the kinds of questions that this book will address. If not all turn out to be answerable in molecular terms as yet, the reader nevertheless will be able to enjoy this molecular quest through the body in health and disease. It is a journey whose path is opposite that into space. What science during the past few hundred years has done is to push the limits of our knowledge of the world in two directions: knowledge of space, where the nearest star is 25 trillion miles away, and knowledge of the molecules that make up all matter in the universe, where a molecule of water is a billion times smaller than the resolution of our eyes.

It is with some of these tiny particles that we are concerned. Not with those that make up rocks and earth, desert and volcanos, but with those that make up plants and microbes, animals and man. In short, with the molecules of life. And it is the molecules within man in particular that are the subject of this book. The most abundant molecule in the body is water, and it is also the most abundant molecule on the surface of the earth. After water, the most abundant molecules within our bodies are proteins. Although some 5000 times larger than a molecule of water, proteins are still far too small to be seen with the naked eye. Even DNA (deoxyribose nucleic acid), which is a molecule some 30,000 times larger than the average protein molecule, is still too small to be seen directly with our eyes. Water, proteins, and DNA are the most important molecules in our body. The other molecules are intermediate in size between water and DNA: They are carbohydrates, fats, and the building blocks of which proteins, nucleic acids, carbohydrates, and fats are made. These building blocks are molecules like amino acids, nucleotides, sugars, and fatty acids. It is the way in which all of these molecules interact with one another in our bodies that is responsible for the function of organs like liver, heart, or brain. And it is when the interactions—our metabolism—go awry, or when the wrong kinds of proteins are made, that disease rears its ugly head. So to understand the workings of our bodies in health and disease at the most fundamental level, it is the nature of the molecules of life that we need to understand. It is here that our journey begins.

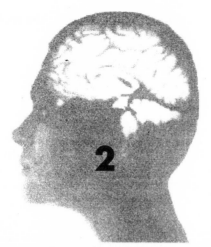

THE MOLECULES OF LIFE

All matter is made up of molecules: the earth on which we live, the water of rivers and the sea, the air we breathe. Matter *is* molecules: molecules of aluminum silicate and other salts in the earth, molecules of water in rivers and the sea, molecules of nitrogen and oxygen in air. Molecules are the smallest particles that have an independent existence; if you took a piece of sugar and were able to cut it up into pieces of ever-decreasing size, you would eventually come to a piece that you could not cut up any more. That piece would be a molecule of sugar. But you would have to halve the original piece a thousand million million million, or 10^{21}, times to get down to one molecule. Now consider a small glass of water. This contains some million million million million, or 10^{24}, molecules of H_2O. If you decided to drink the glass of water, the molecules will eventually pass out of your body and into the sea, by way of sewers and rivers. Over a period of time those 10^{24} molecules will become distributed throughout all of the oceans of the world, by oceanic currents and by evaporation into the atmosphere, to be returned as rain. So if you were then, many years later, to dip that original glass into the sea, whether in San Francisco or

Boston, Rio de Janeiro or Sydney, it would contain some 100 of the original molecules.

Another way to comprehend the smallness of molecules, and the large number that make up matter, is to consider the molecules of nitrogen in Abraham Lincoln's last gasp as he lay dying in Ford's Theater in Washington in 1865. With every breath you now take—whether in Des Moines or Delhi, Montreal or Moscow—you are likely to inhale at least one of those molecules. The mathematically inclined reader may by now have worked out that a molecule of nitrogen is about the same size as a molecule of water, and that a molecule of sugar is bigger, though not by much, just 20-fold larger. Such molecules are therefore much too small to see with even the most powerful microscope ever developed. The size of a molecule of water is around 0.3 nanometer (nm); 1 nm is 10^9 meter (m) or a millionth of the point of a needle. The composition of water as H_2O, or of air as a mixture of nitrogen (N_2) and oxygen (O_2), or of sugar as $C_{12}H_{22}O_{11}$, is based on chemical analysis not of single molecules, but of millions of millions of molecules. The reader should be aware that molecules are made up of atoms—two atoms of hydrogen and one of oxygen in water, two atoms of nitrogen in a molecule of nitrogen, and so forth. Because most atoms do not exist as separate entities, except at extraordinarily high temperatures, it is with molecules that this book—and indeed most of chemistry—is concerned.

The composition of our planet's crust today—whether desert, soil, or rocks—is not so different from what it was some 4 billion years ago. Nearly a billion years before that, when primordial gas and dust emitted from the Sun started to condense into the Earth and the other planets, most of the matter was gaseous hydrogen and helium, as it is still in the Sun today. At the extreme temperatures of the sun, nuclear reactions occur. Unlike chemical reactions, in which the participating atoms remain intact, nuclear reactions involve the change of one atom into another—generally with the release of an enormous amount of energy, as in the atomic or nuclear bomb. The results of nuclear explosions some 4.5 billion years ago created the atoms that have existed on Earth ever since. They produced some 90 different atoms—the elements found on Earth today. The molecules formed by these 90 different atoms exist on Earth today, with one important addition: namely, molecules that are made up of carbon (C), hydrogen (H), and oxygen (O), with lesser amounts of other elements such as nitrogen (N), phosphorus (P), and sulfur (S) being present in some of them. These are the molecules of living matter—molecules like glucose and proteins, RNA and DNA. Together with water, they make up all microbes, plants, and animals.

How did their synthesis from simpler molecules come about? It is, of course, impossible to know exactly what the conditions were on Earth 4 billion years ago; all we can do is guess, by trying to understand what conditions favor the synthesis of such "organic" molecules. The word *organic* was coined in the last century to distinguish the molecules that constitute living matter from the molecules that constitute nonliving, or "inorganic," matter. Organic molecules were known to be complex and to be made up of carbon, hydrogen, oxygen, nitrogen, phosphorus, and sulfur in hundreds of different combinations. Until 1828 it was thought that organic molecules possessed some "vital," i.e., life-related, quality that was absent in inorganic molecules. But in that year the German chemist Friedrich Wöhler (Figure 5) heated ammonium cyanate (NH_4CNO), an inorganic salt of ammonia, and found that he had turned it into urea (NH_2CONH_2), a product found in the urine of certain animals including humans, and hence an organic compound. A decade or so later, acetic acid (CH_3COOH) was synthesized from inorganic molecules. Acetic acid, a constituent of vinegar, is formed if a bottle of wine, containing alcohol (CH_3CH_2OH), is left standing around for too long without its cork: The oxygen in the air oxidizes alcohol to acetic acid. Acetic acid is also formed when fresh orange juice passes its sell-by date: In this case the sugar in the orange juice becomes oxidized to acetic acid without first being fermented to alcohol. These early nineteenth-century experiments synthesizing urea and acetic acid revealed that the distinction between inorganic and organic compounds in terms of some vital force could no longer be sustained.

From many experiments carried out over the last 40 years or so, it seems pretty clear that conditions on the Earth's surface

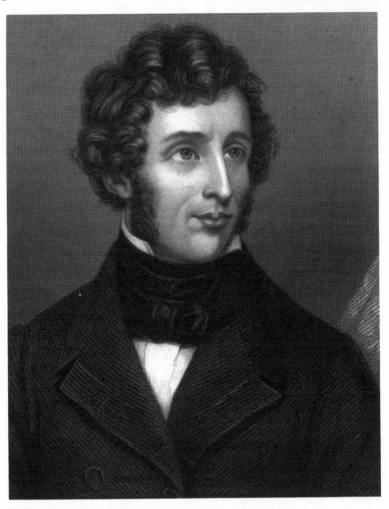

5. Friedrich Wöhler. Sipple engraving by C. Cook after C. L'Allemand. Courtesy of The Wellcome Institute Library, London.

4 billion years ago were not exactly the same as today: The composition of rocks and deserts may have been similar, but the temperature was considerably higher than now and the atmosphere lacked oxygen; nitrogen was present, and more carbon dioxide. Perhaps as a result of lightning, volcanic eruptions, the impact of meteorites, and other brief periods of extreme conditions, cou-

pled with the catalytic effects of certain clays that are present on the earth's crust, the complex array of organic molecules that exist on earth today started to form. And with their formation began the process of life: the evolution of structures that have the unique property of being able to replicate themselves.

What the earliest forms of life were, we do not know. All we can say is that the oldest known fossils are of microbes that appear to be around 4 billion years old; to date no fossils of plants or animals of that age have been found. Estimating the age of fossils and other ancient specimens has been made by carbon dating, a process first introduced by the American scientist Harold Urey (Figure 6) half a century ago, and it is still in use—together

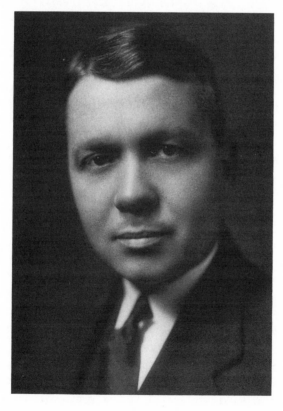

6. Harold Urey. Nobel laureate, 1934. Copyright: The Nobel Foundation, Stockholm.

with more modern techniques—today. One of the most surprising outcomes of analyzing the molecules present in microbes, plants, and animals is that they are all alike. The molecules that make up a staphylococcus or a malarial parasite, a blade of grass or an orchid, an earthworm or a human being, are all remarkably similar. Only by a complete sequence analysis of an organism's DNA can the different forms of life be uniquely distinguished. So similar are the constituent molecules that if one were presented with a homogenized sample of staphylococcus, malarial parasite, blade of grass, orchid, earthworm, or human being, it would be quite difficult to identify the particular form of life by chemical analysis of the constituent molecules alone. In each case there are proteins, nucleic acids like DNA and RNA, carbohydrates, and fats. Yet a second's glance (under a microscope in the case of staphylococcus or malarial parasite) is sufficient to identify a blade of grass, an orchid, an earthworm, or a human being in its intact state.

Not only are the molecules—the chemistry—of all forms of life remarkably similar, but so also is the basic unit of structure: All life is made up of cells. The molecules of living matter, chief of which are water, carbohydrate, fat, proteins, RNA, and DNA, (Figure 7) assemble themselves into the specialized structures we call cells. Every cell has a thin membrane around it; within that sheath most of the molecular interactions that enable life to go on—the oxidation of carbohydrate and fat, the synthesis of proteins, RNA, DNA, and so forth—take place. In the case of plants and animals, cells are grouped together, rather like a honeycomb, to form tissues and organs. It is the pattern that such groups of cells take up in flower, leaf, or stem, in muscle, heart, or brain, that distinguishes plants from animals. The actual size of individual cells is much the same in plants and animals, whether in a blade of grass or a palm tree, in a mosquito or an elephant. That size is around 10 μm (1 μm is a millionth of a meter). Though cells are too small to be seen with the naked eye, they are nonetheless large enough to accommodate many millions of molecules like glucose or water. The one exception to this generalization are the egg cells of animals: These are many times larger than the other cells of the body. Eggs of birds are particularly

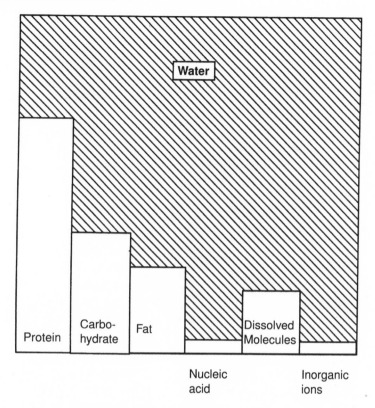

7. Composition of cells. From *An Introduction to Human Biochemistry* by C. A. Pasternak, Oxford University Press, 1979.

large (the size of our breakfast egg is a good example), but even the eggs of amphibians and fish, though much smaller, are still large enough to be seen with the naked eye (and in the case of caviar, eaten with relish). The eggs of sea urchins, which are somewhat smaller, are a delicacy in the Mediterranean; in other countries they are used for research into the early stages of embryonic development (Figure 8).

Microbes, such as bacteria and protozoa, exist as single cells that are generally much smaller than the cells of plants and animals. The mycobacteria that give rise to tuberculosis and leprosy, for example, live within the cells of our lungs and other organs,

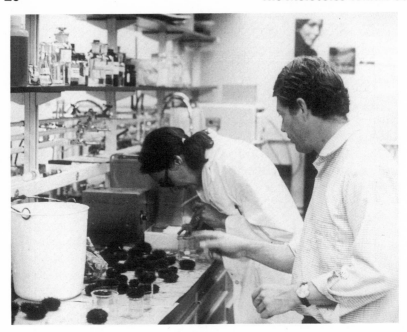

8. Research on sea urchins. The author and Audrey Pasternak in the laboratory of Dr. John O'Brien at the University of California San Diego at La Jolla in 1970.

and the protozoan parasite responsible for malaria multiplies within liver cells and red blood cells. Viruses are smaller still and multiply not only within the cells of animals and plants, but within bacteria and protozoa also; they are not, however, cellular and free-living like bacteria, but require the machinery present in the cells of animals, plants, or microbes to multiply. The recently discovered infectious agents known as prions are smaller yet again: They appear to be made up of nothing more than protein, and like viruses replicate only within cells of another organism; so far they have been isolated only from animals, in which they appear to be responsible for diseases like bovine spongiform encephalitis (BSE) in cattle, scrapie in sheep, and Creutzfeldt–Jakob disease (CJD) in humans.

The fact that all forms of life contain the same molecules and that these form similar structures, namely, cells, leads one to suppose that life arose only once and that it is from some primordial cell that all subsequent organisms are derived (Figure 9). This is the accepted view among the majority of scientists. There is, however, a contrasting view that some forms of life, such as viruses, developed outside our atmosphere and that these have landed on Earth within meteoric dust and have, indeed, contributed to the evolution of the creatures on Earth today. Currently there is also speculation as to whether some form of life ever existed on Mars. If the conditions on Mars at some time mirrored those on Earth, this is a possibility and it would then be fascinating to know what kinds of molecules evolved on that planet. The possibility that they might include infectious microbes is

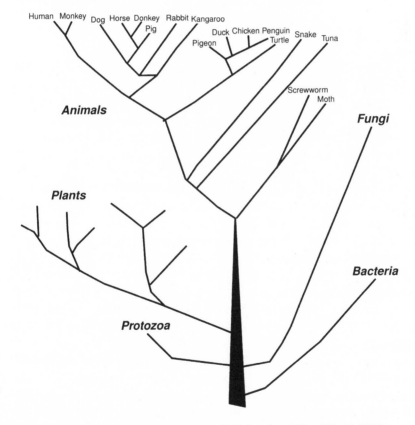

9. Tree of life. Adapted from *Encyclopaedia Brittanica* (15th edition), 1994.

taken so seriously by scientists that when a sample of Martian soil is brought back to Earth by NASA in a mission planned for 2008, it will be treated with as much caution as if it contained viruses as deadly as Ebola. The samples will be brought back in hermetically sealed double containers and will be handled by robots in a specially constructed "Mars" laboratory. If these samples do indeed turn out to contain molecules other than those of rock already identified, they are likely to be made up of carbon atoms in various combinations: for none of the other elements is able to form anything like the millions of different compounds, all based on carbon, that have been found naturally on Earth or have been synthesized in a chemical laboratory. What would be surprising is if molecules found on Mars turn out to be similar in detail to those found on Earth, for that would suggest a common origin: The conditions on Mars are unlikely to have been *exactly* the same as those on Earth 4.5 billion years ago, and they are certainly not the same now. Instead, one might expect the molecules to be different from the glucose, proteins, nucleic acids (DNA and RNA), and so forth that have evolved on Earth. The same speculation, of course, applies to life outside our solar system. Although Earth is probably unique in our solar system in having just the right conditions of temperature, moisture, and so forth to sustain life, there is no reason why such conditions could not prevail on planets in other solar systems. Indeed, given that the galaxy—the Milky Way—of which our solar system is a part, contains around 100 billion other stars, and that there are more than a billion other galaxies in the universe, it would be surprising if events similar to those that led to the formation of life on Earth had *not* occurred elsewhere. Finding them is another matter: The nearest solar system to our own is 4.3 light-years (25×10^{12} miles) away, and it would take a person traveling at current speeds of space flight, 250,000 years, or 6000 generations of human life, to get there.

As already mentioned, organic molecules were originally thought to be produced only by living matter—by plants and microbes and animals. With this distinction having been refuted by Wöhler's experiment showing that an inorganic salt could be turned into an organic molecule, organic molecules are now defined as those made up of carbon atoms, together with varying amounts of hydrogen, oxygen, and other atoms; some of these are found in nature, others are man-made in the laboratory. There are millions of different molecules made up merely of C, H, and O in various proportions. They range from simple molecules to complicated ones: simple molecules like carbon dioxide (CO_2), methane (CH_4)—a gas that is formed by microbes at the bottom of stagnant ponds and is thought to have been much more plentiful in prebiotic times—and methanol [CH_3OH, wood alcohol; not to be confused with ethanol (C_2H_5OH), the alcohol of hard liquor, wine, and beer; drinking wood alcohol causes blindness]; and complicated molecules like cholesterol ($C_{27}H_{46}O$)—discussed in later chapters—and carotene ($C_{40}H_{56}$), the orange ingredient of carrots that can be broken down in the body to vitamin A ($C_{20}H_{30}O$), which is important in the prevention of night blindness.

The reason why there are so many molecules made up of carbon is as follows. Atoms bond to each other in defined patterns: H forms only one bond, O forms two, N forms three, but C is unique in forming four bonds (Figure 10). Consequently, carbon atoms are able to form extensive, three-dimensional molecules. The nature of the bonds that hold atoms together is too complicated to go into detail here. The American scientist Linus Pauling (Figure 11), a Nobel laureate first for Chemistry and then for Peace—better known for his crusade to persuade us to take vitamin C, an ingredient of orange juice, against the common cold—wrote an entire treatise on the subject of the chemical bond. Suffice it to say that all atoms are made up of a positively charged nucleus that is surrounded by a number of negatively charged electrons; when two atoms approach close enough so that two of their electrons can somehow be shared between them, a bond is formed. This is because the total energy of the system is less when atoms are bonded, than when they are unbonded, and all systems tend to take up the forms that have the least energy. Consider a coiled metal spring: If you compress it, it gains energy; if you now release it, it jumps back to its original size by a release of energy. This is roughly how our muscles work: If energy is supplied (ultimately through the oxidation of foodstuffs as described below),

a) Covalent Bonds

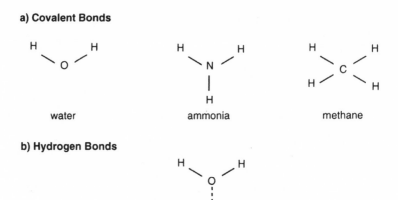

b) Hydrogen Bonds

10. Atoms, bonds, and molecules.

the fibers contract; when the source of energy is removed, the muscle fibers relax back to their original length. Because of the sharing nature of the chemical bond it has been termed a covalent bond: "co" for the sharing aspect and "valent" for the number of bonds formed by different atoms (1 for H, 2 for O, 3 for N, and 4 for C). A covalent bond is stronger than a hydrogen bond (described below) in which only one electron is shared between two atoms (Figure 10). The third type of bond that occurs in molecules—particularly in inorganic ones—is the ionic bond.

Ions occur for the following reason. We have seen that atoms like hydrogen, oxygen, nitrogen, and carbon tend to share their electrons with a neighboring atom. This forms the covalent bonds that hold the atoms together in molecules as simple as methane (CH_4) or as complicated as cholesterol ($C_{27}H_{46}O$). Hydrogen is an exceptional atom in that it also has a tendency to lose an electron entirely, to become a positively charged hydrogen ion, H^+. When this happens, say in a molecule of water (H–O–H), the electron lost by H is taken up by its neighbor, O, to form a negatively charged ion, OH^-. Water, in fact, is a mixture of H_2O, H^+, and OH^-. H_2O accounts for more than 99%, with only 0.00001% each as H^+ and OH^-. This is because ions of opposite

c) More complicated molecules

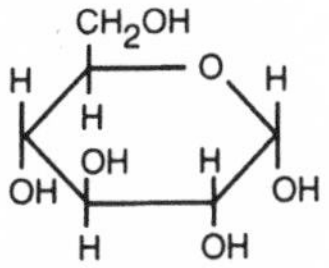

glucose (a sugar)

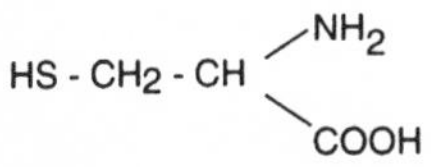

cysteine (an amino acid)

$CH_3 - CH_2 - CH_2 - CH_2 - CH_2 - CH_2 - CH_2 - CH_2 - CH_2 - CH_2 - CH_2 - CH_2 - CH_2 - CH_2 - CH_2 - CH_2 - CH_2 - COOH$

stearic acid (saturated fatty acid)

$CH_3 - CH_2 - CH_2 - CH_2 - CH_2 - CH_2 - CH_2 - CH_2 - CH = CH - CH_2 - CH_2 - CH_2 - CH_2 - CH_2 - CH_2 - CH_2 - COOH$

oleic acid (unsaturated fatty acid)

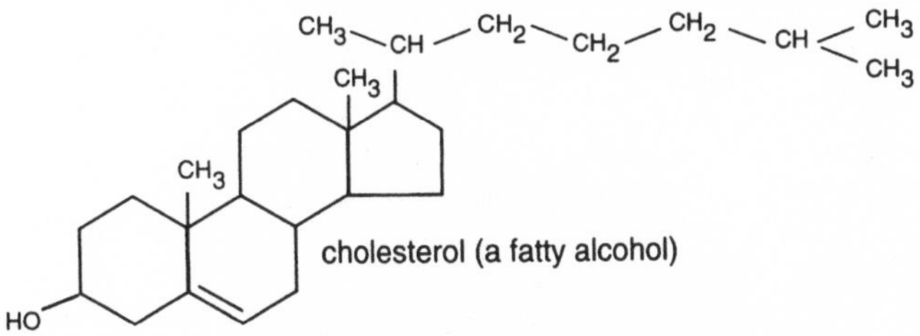

cholesterol (a fatty alcohol)

10. (*continued*)

charge attract each other, just as the north end of one magnet is attracted to the south end of another. The result is that H^+ and OH^- readily combine to become H–O–H. The attraction between positive and negative has been extended to explain the attraction between male and female, but as is evident to all, there are too many cases of like attracting like to make this argument a tenable one: Whatever the attractive stimulus between people—whether shape of face or sexual organs, body odor or quality of mind— the molecular nature of what attracts one person to another has yet to be worked out. Nevertheless, it is used as an illustration for the ionic bond in Figure 12 (below). Depending on whether there is a slight excess of H^+ or OH^-, liquids are said to be either acid or alkaline. Keen gardeners who measure the acidity or alkalinity of their soil are aware of the scale—known as pH—used to measure this. At neutrality, the pH is 7. If the pH is 6 the solution is slightly acid, whereas at pH 8 it is slightly alkaline. The strongest solutions of acid approach a pH of 0 and the strongest solutions

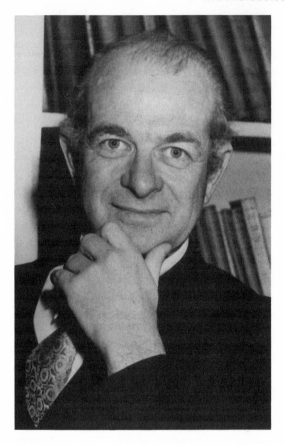

11. Linus Pauling. Nobel laureate, 1954 and 1962. Copyright: The Nobel Foundation, Stockholm.

of alkali, a pH of 14. The pH of our blood, as well as the pH inside all cells, is around 7. Only in the stomach does the pH fall as low as 2 via secretion of strong hydrochloric acid (HCl) from specialized cells lining the stomach wall; the urine is also acid, with a pH of between 4.5 and 7. The tendency to form ions is particularly strong in atoms like sodium (Na) and chlorine (Cl). In fact, sodium chloride (chlorine is the name given only to the free atom or to a molecule of chlorine gas, Cl_2)—common salt (NaCl)—is made up *entirely* of Na^+ (formed by loss of one electron from Na) and Cl^- (formed by gain of one electron by Cl).

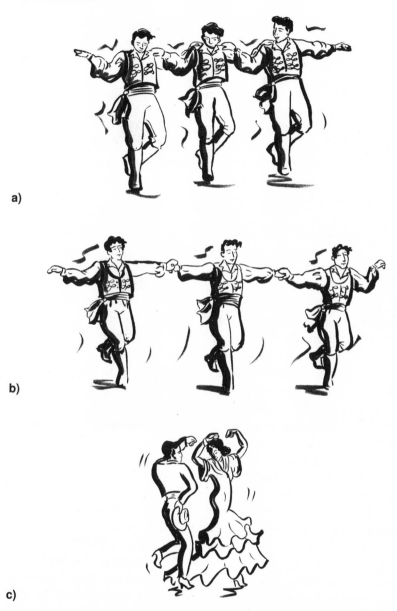

12. Human bonds. (a) Dancers linking arms, representing strong, covalent bonds; (b) dancers holding hands, representing weaker, longer, hydrogen bonds; (c) attraction between male and female, representing ionic bonds. Drawn by Denise Young, St. George's Hospital Medical School, London.

The hydrogen atom is exceptional for another reason. It also forms a bond that is halfway between a covalent bond and an ionic bond, by sharing its electron (it has only one) with a neighboring atom such as O or N that has a tendency (like Cl) to attract electrons. That bond, which is unique to hydrogen, is appropriately called a hydrogen or H bond. Figure 12 illustrates in human terms the three bond types discussed here. The strength of a covalent bond is illustrated by the strength of the link created when each member of a group of Greek dancers—or the ladies of the Folies Bergère doing the cancan—links arms. The link between adjacent members of the group is stronger than if they merely hold hands. This is the difference between a covalent bond and a hydrogen bond. The analogy is appropriate because a hydrogen bond is longer than a covalent bond.

In order to understand how our body works we need to know the properties of the molecules within us. The most abundant molecules that contain only C, H, and O are **fats** and **carbohydrates.** Together with protein they are the main energy-yielding constituents of our diet and they serve as an energy reserve in the body; fat alone accounts for 80% of this reserve. The major fat molecule in food and the body is triglyceride, so called because it is composed of three chains of fatty acid linked to glycerol. Triglyceride is concentrated in cells—adipocytes or adipose (fat) cells—that lie just under the skin. As might be expected, obese people have many more adipose cells than do lean people. Fats like triglyceride are typically greasy substances that exist in adipose cells in the form of fat droplets.

Carbohydrate occurs in the diet in two forms. One is as small molecules like glucose (containing 6 carbon atoms) or sucrose, the sugar of sugar beet and sugarcane (containing 12 carbon atoms). The other is as large molecules that contain many thousands of glucose residues; large molecules that are made up of multiples of simpler units are called polymers (which we shall meet again in proteins and the nucleic acids, DNA and RNA). The chemical synthesis of a polymer made from formaldehyde and phenol by the American chemist Leo Baekeland (originally a Belgian) in 1909 was one of the greatest technological advances of this century: It gave us our first plastic, Bakelite, named for its inventor. The United States quickly became the leader in the industry. During the 1930s scientists at E. I. du Pont de Nemours revolutionized the clothing industry through the manufacture of nylon fibers from polyamides. To return to carbohydrates, the small molecules are found to any degree only in plants—sugarcane and sugar beet are virtually pure sucrose—whereas polymers of glucose are found in both animals and plants: In animals the polymer is a highly branched molecule, glycogen, whereas in plants the polymer is a much less branched molecule, starch. Plants contain a third polymer of glucose, cellulose, that is abundant in leaves and grass. Because the structure of cellulose is slightly different from that of glycogen and starch, animals—including man—cannot degrade cellulose. For animals such as cattle, sheep, or horses that virtually live off grass, it is not the enzymes (discussed below) of these animals that degrade the cellulose; instead it is the enzymes of symbiotic bacteria (meaning living in harmony) that dwell in the stomach and intestines of their host, that turn the cellulose into products (largely fatty acids and glucose) that are easily absorbed and utilized by the animal host. So important is this process that cattle, for example, have four stomachs, each filled with cellulose-degrading bacteria. If we were prepared to colonize our gut with such bacteria, we too might be able to live off grass, though the odor of our breath associated with by-products of the bacterial degradation of celluluse might put some people off. The carbohydrate that is absorbed by animals—whether ruminant or man—is stored as granules of glycogen in muscle and liver; small amounts are present in other tissues.

The main distinction between fats and carbohydrates is that fats do not dissolve in water, whereas carbohydrates—at least those with only 6 or 12 carbon atoms—do. This is an important difference and organic molecules are classified as either insoluble in water or soluble in water. Insoluble molecules are hydrophobic (water-hating) whereas water-soluble molecules are hydrophilic (water-loving). Fats are hydrophobic, but carbohydrates are hydrophilic. Some molecules, like the **phospholipids** that constitute a protective sheath or membrane around every cell in our body, are both hydrophobic and hydrophilic; that is, one part of the molecule is able to dissolve in water (by making hydrogen bonds with the oxygen atoms of water) while the other part has no affinity for water. Some people regard phospholipids as being neither water-soluble nor fat-soluble, and use the term amphipathic, whereas for those who regard them in the opposite sense, the term amphiphilic applies. This difference may be likened to that between a pessimist and an optimist: The pessimist sees a half-filled glass as "half-empty," whereas the optimist sees it as "half-full."

The hydrophobic parts of phospholipids tend to associate with each other, and the hydrophilic parts tend to associate with water. Because of this, phospholipids form two types of structure: spheres, called vesicles, in which the hydrophilic parts point outward and make contact with water while the hydrophobic parts point inward and make contact with totally hydrophobic lipids like triglyceride; or sheets made up of two layers of phospholipid molecules in which the hydrophilic parts of each point outward and make contact with water while the hydrophobic parts point inward and make contact with each other, as illustrated in Figure 13. The fat droplets that are present in milk, or in the blood after a fatty meal, are vesicles; the membranes surrounding cells are double-layered sheets. Detergents that are used for washing clothes are akin to phospholipids in that each molecule has both a hydrophobic and a hydrophilic part. Thus, detergents are able to associate both with fats and with water, as a result of which they are able to dissolve grease stains very effectively.

We have seen that glycogen and starch are polymers made up of thousands of glucose units. Two other types of polymer are even more important constituents of man, as well as of all other living organisms: proteins and nucleic acids (DNA and RNA). Unlike glycogen and triglyceride, which are found only in specialized cells like those of muscle, liver, or adipose tissue, **proteins** are found in all cells of the body, for their presence is crucial to the life of every cell. It is to be noted that while adipose cells, for example, are distinctive in making and storing triglyceride, they are not restricted to any particular organ, but occur all over the body. The same is true of muscle cells: While they synthesize specific proteins like actin and myosin that are responsible for muscle contraction, they too are found all over the body—in the heart, in

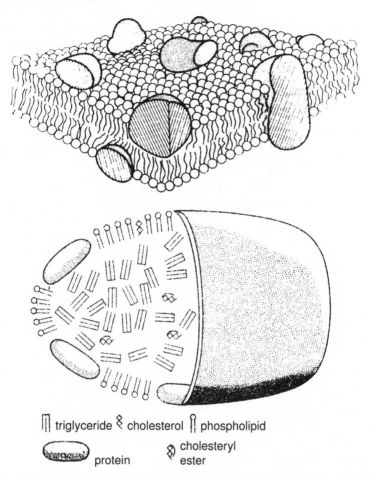

|| triglyceride ⅄ cholesterol ⨆ phospholipid

protein   cholesteryl ester

13. Phospholipids. (Top) Bilayer. A double layer of phospholipid, with proteins embedded in it. (Bottom) Vesicle. A single layer of phospholipid, plus cholesterol and protein, surrounds a mixture of triglyceride and cholesteryl ester (cholesterol linked to fatty acid). From *An Introduction to Human Biochemistry* by C. A. Pasternak, Oxford University Press, 1979.

skeletal muscle that moves our limbs, and in smooth muscle; smooth muscle cells line the blood vessels to make them elastic and in the stomach and intestine they enable these organs to carry out the rhythmic movements that push food along as it is being degraded. In fact, actin and myosin, together with another protein (collagen) that is present *outside* cells and that we shall return to in

Chapter 9, make up the bulk of protein in our body: All three fulfill essentially a structural role. The other function of proteins is to act as biological catalysts (enzymes), as will be described below. Suffice it to say here that it is structural proteins and enzymes that give an organism its distinct features. The enzymes within flower, leaf, and stem, within muscle, heart, and liver, each promote different molecular interactions (as well as many common ones). The result of those interactions is the formation of specific molecules—carbohydrates and fats as well as other proteins—that give each organ a distinct molecular menu that underlies its shape and, in the case of plants, its color. Thus, it is ultimately the different proteins within buttercup, sunflower, or orchid, within earthworm, elephant, or man, that give the resultant organisms their characteristic differences. At this stage the reader should simply consider proteins to be polymers of small molecules, similar in size to glucose, called amino acids. All amino acids contain one or more nitrogen atoms in addition to carbon, hydrogen, and oxygen; some also have sulfur. Proteins are made up of long chains of amino acids linked together; there are no branches. Different combinations of just 20 different amino acids make up all of the 100,000 or so different proteins in our body. It is the sequence in which the different amino acids are linked together that distinguishes one protein from another. The size of proteins varies according to the number of amino acids of which it is composed: A typical protein might contain some 100 amino acids, and therefore be 100 times larger than an amino acid.

DNA and RNA are, like proteins, found in virtually every cell of the body. The function of **DNA** is to act as a reservoir of information: It specifies the exact structure of every protein in our body. DNA, which is the same in every cell, is doubled each time a cell divides, and is passed on intact from generation to generation. The role of **RNA** is to decode specific parts of the information contained within DNA so as to translate that information into proteins. In short, DNA makes RNA and RNA makes proteins. Our red blood cells (also called erythrocytes) contain no DNA or RNA, and thus are unable to multiply or to synthesize proteins. Nevertheless they have a very important function, that of transporting oxygen throughout the body. Oxygen is concentrated within the red blood cell by binding to the protein hemoglobin. Since red cells lack the machinery for making proteins, hemoglobin is synthesized in a precursor cell, called a reticulocyte, that loses its RNA—specific for hemoglobin—when it matures into a red blood cell. It is in the precursor cell of a reticulocyte, called an erythroblast, that hemoglobin-specific RNA is made from DNA; as the erythroblast matures into a reticulocyte (see Figure 44 in Chapter 5), it loses all of its DNA. Such a progression of ever-increasing specificity of function is typical of the way that all of the body's specialized cells—be they muscle, adipose, or nerve cell—mature; the difference is that in none of those cases is the DNA and the ability to make proteins, lost. The essential part of a molecule of hemoglobin is an iron atom that binds oxygen (see Figure 35 in Chapter 4), and this is the reason why blood is red (iron is red whether in ferrous rocks or in hemoglobin). The redness is particularly marked in hemoglobin that has just picked up its oxygen from the lungs, as will be described in the following chapter. It is less red—almost blue—in blood that has passed through the body and is on its way back to the lungs.

DNA and RNA resemble proteins in being polymers of small molecules joined together in a long chain. In this instance the small molecules that make up the polymer are not amino acids, but nucleotides—deoxyribonucleotides in the case of DNA, and ribonucleotides in the case of RNA. A nucleotide is a molecule composed of a nitrogen-containing compound, a sugar, and a phosphoric acid residue (referred to as phosphate for short, as in ammonium phosphate, the fertilizer that makes lawns grow). In DNA the sugar is deoxyribose; in RNA it is ribose. There are four nitrogen-containing compounds in DNA and the same number in RNA. Those in DNA are adenine, guanine, cytosine, and thymine, and those in RNA are adenine, guanine, cytosine, and uracil; the structure of these molecules is shown in Figure 60 in Chapter 7. For simplicity we shall refer to the different nucleotides in DNA as A, G, C, and T and those in RNA as A, G, C, and U. Because nucleotides contain a phosphate residue that is acid, the two types of compounds are called deoxyribonucleic acid and ribonucleic acid, respectively, *nucleic* indicating that DNA is found in the nucleus of cells. Although RNA is found both in the nucleus and in the surrounding fluid (cytoplasm) of a cell, it is synthesized only in the nucleus.

The function of DNA, then, is to store the entire genetic information of an individual organism and to pass this on every time a cell divides to form two daughter cells. What is this genetic information? It is the ability of a stretch of DNA, called a gene, to synthesize a complementary stretch of RNA; complementary in that it is the same length as a gene, but that every A in DNA is replaced in RNA by U, every G by C, every C by G, and every T by A. Such a molecule of RNA then goes on to form a particular protein as described below. The proteins of buttercups and orchids, of earthworms and elephants, are different because the sequence of the four nucleotides (A, G, C, T) in their respective genes is different. To put it another way: if every nucleotide is represented by a different colored bead—say Amber, Green, Cream, and Turquoise—strung on an immensely long piece of twine, then the sequence of colors along the twine would represent the different sequences of nucleotides along a gene. By looking at a mixture of such long necklaces thrown together, it would be very difficult indeed to tell one apart from another. Only by carefully analyzing the exact sequence in which Amber, Green, Cream, and Turquoise beads are linked together could one tell one necklace apart from another. So it is with genes. The properties of one stretch of DNA are so like the properties of another that one cannot tell them apart by simple chemical analysis. Only by careful determination of the exact sequence of A, G, C, and T along the stretch of DNA can one gene be distinguished from another.

How does the RNA corresponding to a particular gene determine the sequence of amino acids in a protein? Every three nucleotides in RNA specify a particular amino acid in a protein: CGC (a triplet of Cream, Green, and Cream beads in the above example), codes for the amino acid alanine, AAT (a triplet of Amber, Amber, and Turquoise) codes for the amino acid leucine, and so on. The length of a protein is therefore proportional to the length of the RNA that specifies that protein, and hence to the length of the gene that specifies the RNA. In fact, genes are not discrete molecules like the proteins for which they code. They are themselves linked, gene to gene, along the entire length of a chromosome. It is chromosomes that are discrete units, i.e., discrete giant molecules of DNA. Despite the fact that chromosomes are the largest molecules in our bodies, and indeed in the whole living world, they are still much less than a tenth of the size of a cell in which they reside. Humans contain 23 different chromosomes that vary in size and hence in genetic content; each cell in the human body contains the same number of chromosomes—actually 46 since they are present in pairs (Figure 14). Closely related species have similar numbers

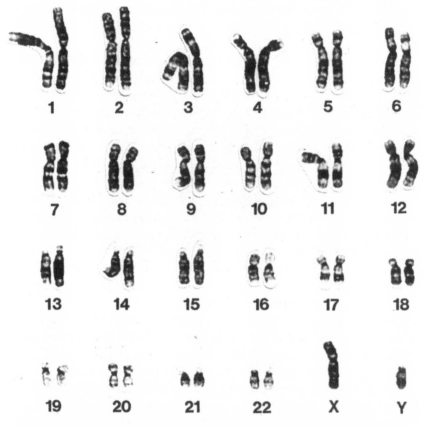

14. Chromosomes. The chromosomes of a male. A female has the same pairs of chromosomes 1–22, but two copies of the X chromosome instead of an X and a Y. From *Biochemistry for the Medical Sciences* by S. J. Higgins, A. J. Turner, and E. J. Wood, Longman Scientific and Technical, 1994, reprinted by permission of Addison Wesley Longman Ltd.

of chromosomes: chimpanzees, which incidentally are closer in their genetic makeup to humans than to orangutans, have 24 chromosomes to our 23; mice have 20, and so on. Another reason why DNA is so much longer than proteins is that only some 10% of it corresponds to genes; the remaining 90% of DNA is nongenetic. This includes stretches near every gene that control the expression of that gene. In other words, such a region of DNA causes the adjacent gene to be switched on and copied into its complementary RNA. This is achieved by specific proteins that "sense" the conditions in a cell and whether a particular protein needs to be made or not. Then, by binding to a part of the control region of DNA, the sensor protein somehow switches on the synthesis of the RNA complementary to the gene in question. As soon as that RNA is made, it is translated into its corresponding protein. Other nongenetic regions of DNA have other functions. Some stretches code for types of RNA that are *not* translated into proteins. Other stretches have roles that we do not yet understand.

The DNA in a chromosome is very long indeed. If stretched out it would be some 5 cm (2 inches) long; yet the size of the nucleus in cells, in which DNA resides most of the time, is around 1 μm (= 0.0001 cm) or less. Hence, DNA is folded, coiled, and wound around itself to such an extent that its length is reduced some 50,000-fold (Figure 15). It is equivalent to compressing a 10-mile-long piece of thread into a 1-square-foot box. As mentioned above, all cells have roughly the same size. Never, therefore, is DNA fully unwound. Indeed, it has never been fully unwound since cells first evolved some 4 billion years ago, as the cells of our microbial ancestors were probably no bigger than ours are today. Yet every time a cell divides, its entire length of DNA is somehow copied with virtually 100% accuracy. And every time a molecule of a protein, such as hemoglobin, is synthesized, a precise region of that DNA, corresponding to no more than 0.002% of its length, is specifically selected, partially unwound, and copied into its complementary RNA, which is then translated into a protein molecule. RNA and proteins are also folded and coiled in cells, but nothing like the extent to which DNA is coiled. The reduction in length of a protein like hemoglobin, for example, is around 100-fold, not 50,000-fold.

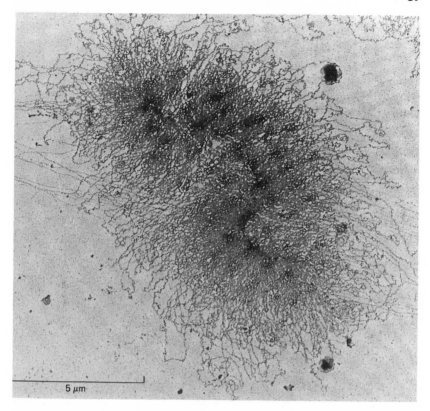

15. Folding of DNA. A single chromatid (one of the two arms of a chromosome; see Figure 14) during mitosis (cell division) of an insect (*Oncopeltus*) cell. It has been visualized by electron microscopy. The chromatid consists of one continuous piece of DNA, folded and coiled back on itself thousands of times. From *Molecular Biology of the Cell* (Fig. 8-23) by B. Alberts, D. Bray, J. Lewis, M. Raff, K. Roberts, and J. D. Watson, Garland Publishing Inc., 1983, with permission.

By what mechanism are molecules like DNA, RNA, and protein folded and why do they remain in the folded state? One of the main reasons for remaining folded is that parts of the molecule have a tendency to interact with other parts of the same molecule through the formation of bonds that keep the resulting folded structure in place. Imagine a long piece of string that has glue applied to it at intervals along its length; assume that the glued portions are able to stick to other glued portions (but not to unglued portions). Now imagine throwing the string into the air and letting it fall onto a surface. By repeating the process a few times, the string will eventually adopt a structure—much smaller than its length—that is kept in place by the glue–glue interactions. That is precisely how proteins (and to a lesser extent DNA and RNA) adopt a highly folded structure. What is the nature of the glue, i.e., the nature of the bonds? One of the most important bonds that contributes to the folded structure of proteins is the hydrogen (H) bond. In contrast to the covalent bonds mentioned earlier, hydrogen bonds are very weak. The reason they are able to maintain the folded structure of a protein is that there are very many of them. H bonds form between atoms like O and N (of which there are a great number in proteins and nucleic acids), to produce O.H.N, O.H.O, and N.H.N whenever these three atoms are sufficiently close to each other and in the right configuration. In the case of a molecule like water (H_2O) in its liquid state, a H bond can form between the O of one molecule and the H of a suitably placed neighbor (Figure 10); when water is in its solid state (i.e., ice), essentially all molecules are linked by H bonds, producing crystalline arrays such as those seen in a snowflake under magnification. Small molecules like glucose, which has five –OH bonds, or those with –OH- and –NH-containing amino acids on the surface of a folded protein, are able to make many H bonds with water. It is this ability that makes glucose and many proteins soluble in water. Fats like triglyceride or cholesterol do not have sufficient O atoms to make H bonds with water, and hence are insoluble in water.

Because the folded state of proteins is crucial to their function as biological catalysts, the H bond is crucial to all forms of life. It plays an even more fundamental role in the structures of RNA and DNA: more fundamental in that it is currently thought that RNA evolved before proteins and that the very earliest forms of life somehow functioned—albeit very slowly—without any proteins at all in what has been dubbed an "RNA world." The role that the H bond plays in nucleic acids is as follows. First, we know that a molecule of DNA in a chromosome is not, in fact, a single long strand of nucleotides, but two such strands. The two strands are held together by H bonds that link every nucleotide on one strand to a nucleotide on the other strand: Because the two strands assume a helical configuration, the structure is referred to as a double helix (Figure 16). H bonds hold the two strands together as follows: Every A on one strand is bonded to a T on the other; every G is bonded to a C, every C to a G, and every T to an A. In short, A is always linked with T, and G is always linked with C. In this way, the "fit"—through H bonding— between A and T is better than between A and either G or C, and that between G and C is better than between G and either A or T. On this difference of fit depends the whole of heredity. For every time a cell divides, its DNA is accurately copied into two daughter molecules of DNA. To achieve this, the two complementary

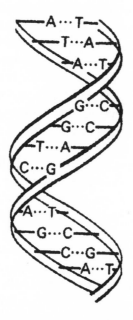

16. DNA double helix. A short portion of the two strands of the DNA backbone (made up of alternate deoxyribose and phosphate residues) are shown as continuous solid lines. The A, T, G, and C residues are shown attached to the DNA backbone by covalent bonds (solid lines) and to each other by hydrogen bonds (dotted lines). From *An Introduction to Human Biochemistry* by C. A. Pasternak, Oxford University Press, 1979.

strands of DNA partially unwind; each strand is then copied into a new complementary strand through H bonding as described above. Imagine two ropes, one black and one white, coiled around each other as in the two strands of DNA. The black and white ropes are complementary to each other in just the way the two strands of DNA are. The coiled ropes begin to unwind and the black rope begins to be copied into a white one, while the white one begins to be copied into a black one. At the end of the process there will be two identical black-and-white ropes; each contains one of the original strands and one newly synthesized one. This is precisely the way that DNA is copied.

The way that a specific region of DNA, namely, a gene, is "read" to produce the protein coded by that gene, is as follows. First, a molecule of complementary RNA is made as described earlier. The mechanism is essentially that described for the copying of a daughter strand of DNA. This complementary RNA molecule, called messenger RNA, is then translated into a protein, using the triplet code mentioned above so as to link specific amino acids in the sequence specified by the DNA of the gene. The process is complicated and involves two other types of complementary RNA (ribosomal RNA and transfer RNA) that are part of the nongenetic regions of DNA. Despite the complexity of the process, some thousands of protein molecules are synthesized within the space of a few minutes. It will now be clear to the reader why elucidation of the structure of DNA—by Francis Crick, James Watson, and the almost forgotten Maurice Wilkins (Figure 17) in the 1950s—is sometimes referred to as the greatest biological discovery of this century; that of the last century was formulating the theory of natural selection to explain the origin of species by Charles Darwin (Figure 18). Life as we know it would not have evolved over the past 4 billion years had conditions not been favorable to the formation and maintenance of H bonds: Those conditions are temperatures between -20°C (-4°F) and 60°C (140°F)—since H bonds are not stable at higher temperatures—and the presence of water.

Triglyceride, glycogen, proteins, DNA, and RNA, then, are the main organic molecules found in cells. In addition, there are lesser amounts of the precursor molecules or building blocks

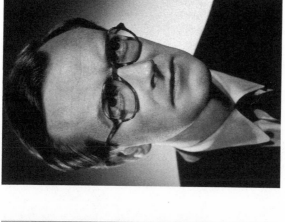
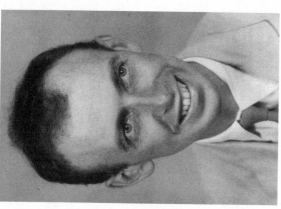
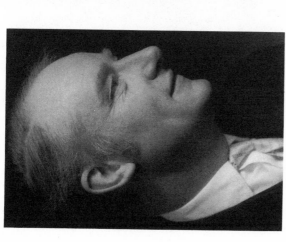

17. Francis Crick, James Watson, and Maurice Wilkins. Nobel laureates, 1962. Rosalind Franklin and Maurice Wilkins provided the X-ray photographs of DNA, from which James Watson and Francis Crick deduced its structure. Edwin Chargaff had shown earlier that in DNA, total A = total T and total G = total C. Left to right: Crick, Watson, and Wilkins. Copyright: The Nobel Foundation, Stockholm.

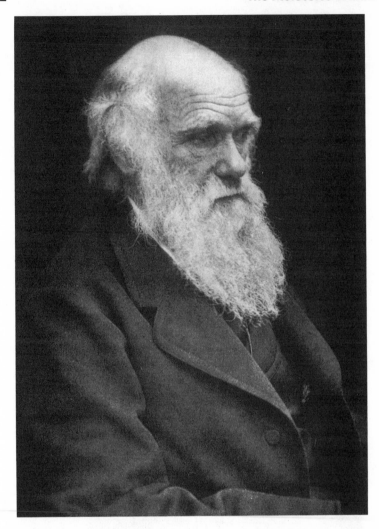

18. Charles Darwin. Photogravure courtesy of The Wellcome Institute Library, London.

from which triglyceride, glycogen, proteins, DNA, and RNA are made; these are fatty acids and glycerol, glucose, amino acids, and nucleotides, as well as a host of related compounds that have a role in the energy metabolism of cells. The actual number of each of these molecules present in a cell is approximately the inverse of its size. A human white blood cell, for example, may contain 46 molecules of DNA (1 molecule per each of the 23 different chromosomes present as pairs), some 10,000 to 100,000 molecules of different proteins and RNA, up to some 100 million molecules of small molecules such as glucose, and a trillion molecules of water.

An apple falling off a tree, or a boy tobogganing his sled down a snowy slope, requires little energy. But the boy pulling his sled back up the slope requires a great deal of energy. Where does this energy come from, and how is it utilized to enable the boy to pull his sled up the hill? The source of all energy on Earth is ultimately the sun, as it is the rays of the sun that enable plants to carry out photosynthesis, i.e., the formation of carbohydrate ($C_6H_{12}O_6$) and other organic molecules from carbon dioxide (CO_2) and water (H_2O). All animals, whether carnivore like lion and leopard, or herbivore like deer and cow, or omnivore like ape and man, depend ultimately on eating plants like grass or the leaves and fruits of shrubs and trees, all of which contain carbohydrate. This is because the food chain of all animals ultimately ends with eating plants. If the synthesis of carbohydrate from CO_2 and H_2O requires energy, then it might be presumed that the reverse process releases energy, and this is indeed correct. The two processes involve a fourth molecule, namely, oxygen (O_2): The synthesis of carbohydrate from carbon dioxide and water gives off oxygen, while oxygen is required to degrade carbohydrate to carbon dioxide and water. The oxidation of carbohydrate (i.e., its degradation by oxygen), then, releases energy. But energy is not a piece of matter—like an apple or a molecule of glucose—that can be caught, stored, and utilized in some way. In order to utilize the energy released during the oxidation of carbohydrate, that process—like any other chemical reaction—has somehow to be coupled to an energy-requiring reaction, as explained below. In the absence of such an energy-requiring reaction, the energy is simply "lost" as heat. The same is true of the apple falling off the tree or the boy tobogganing down the slope (each of which releases potential energy: potential in the sense that if the apple stays on the tree or the boy at the top of the slope, the energy is not released). All forms of energy can be converted into heat (light energy concentrated by a magnifying glass onto a piece of paper and igniting it is a good example), but heat can only partially be converted back into other forms of energy. These generalizations form part of the principles of thermodynamics. The first law of thermodynamics states that the total amount of energy—in whatever form—in a closed or totally isolated system is constant: Since Earth cannot be considered a closed system because light from the sun continually falls on it, the energy associated with it is not constant. The second law states that all closed systems tend to become more and more randomized; again not true of life on Earth, where the exact opposite—an increasing complexity of molecular structure—occurs, again driven by the light from the sun.

Where, then, does the energy to enable the boy to pull his sled back up the slope come from? As mentioned above, all animals, including man, derive their energy from eating other animals or plants. It does not matter which, because both animals and most plants contain carbohydrate. They also contain protein and fat, both of which constitute an alternative energy source. Small molecules like fatty acid, glucose, and amino acids are present in too small an amount in most foods to constitute a major energy source. The other constituents of plants and animals, namely, water (more than 60% of all living matter is water) and inorganic ions like sodium, potassium, calcium, chloride, phosphate, and so forth, do not constitute a source of energy. It is carbohydrate, fat, and protein that release the major source of energy when oxidized by oxygen. The importance of oxygen cannot be over emphasized: Deprivation of oxygen results in death within minutes; deprivation of water results in death within days; deprivation of food results in death within weeks or months. These figures relate to the relative amount of oxygen, water, and food stored in the body. There is virtually no store of oxygen: The red blood cells may concentrate oxygen by binding it to hemoglobin, but their capacity is minute compared with requirement. That is why oxygen has to be rapidly supplied if the heart begins to fail and is therefore unable to push blood around the body fast enough, or if the pressure of air in the cabin of an airplane at

35,000 feet suddenly fails and the air in the cabin is just that of the very "thin" air outside it (the concentration of oxygen in air, namely, 20%, is the same at 35,000 feet as at sea level; what is different is the atmospheric pressure, which is only a quarter of that at sea level; at such low pressures very little oxygen is absorbed by the lungs, leading to a deficit in blood).

The organs most vulnerable to lack of oxygen are heart and brain; although brain accounts for only 2% of body weight, 20% of the circulation—supplying oxygen and glucose—passes through the brain. A parachutist who jumps out of a plane at 35,000 feet and immediately pulls his rip cord will pass out—and is likely to die—long before he hits the ground, because by drifting slowly down to earth he will not lose height quickly enough. The trick, should one find oneself blown out of a plane at 35,000 feet and lucky enough to be wearing a parachute, is to wait until one has dropped some 20,000 feet before pulling the rip cord. This actually happened to a pilot, who survived because he *calculated*—in midair—how long it would take him to fall a sufficient distance (remembering that gravity was pulling him down at 32 feet/second) before it was safe to pull his rip cord. Readers of this book are advised to take it with them when they travel! Another way a person may pass out and die because of lack of oxygen is by compression of the carotid arteries, found on each side of the neck, that supply oxygenated blood from heart to brain. We have all seen movies in which someone is rendered unconscious by an attacker coming up from behind and throwing his arm around the victim's neck: Depending on the skill with which the attacker is able to compress the carotid arteries, he will leave his opponent breathless, passed out, or dead. (The writer was lucky, when attacked by a mugger from behind in the manner described, on a dark night in London a few years ago, to merely pass out and fracture his ankle; his knowledge of biochemistry—gleaned over the preceding 40 years—was not lost, but his wallet was.) Despite such exotic ways by which an insufficiency of oxygen may affect crucial organs of the body, it is a failing heart—unable to pump oxygenated blood to the brain and the rest of the body—that is the most common form of death. Either way, there is no doubt that oxygen is our most important nutrient. Indeed, one of the reasons for our belief that plants emerged before animals during evolution is that without the oxygen generated by plants, no animal could have existed.

Mention has been made on several occasions to the function of proteins as enzymes, or biological catalysts. What is catalysis, and how do enzymes work? In principle, all reactions that are accompanied by a loss of energy occur spontaneously. The oxidation of glucose, one of the major energy-yielding reactions in the body, is a good example:

$$C_6H_{12}O_6 \ + \ 6O_2 \longrightarrow 6CO_2 \ + \ 6H_2O + energy$$
(carbohydrate) (oxygen) (carbon dioxide) (water)

However, if we place some glucose on a spoon and hold it in the air, no reaction occurs. Strictly speaking, this is not quite true: A tiny amount of glucose *is* oxidized to carbon dioxide and water, but it is far too small an amount to measure, and it would take thousands of years for all of the glucose to be oxidized. Yet if we place a flame below the spoon so that it becomes extremely hot, the reaction will be accelerated and the glucose will burn up to carbon dioxide and water. How does this occur? For molecules to interact they have to bump into each other; at room temperature the rate at which oxygen molecules bump into glucose molecules is too slow for reaction to occur. But as molecules are heated up they move faster and faster, so there is a greater chance of making contact and initiating a reaction. The heat that has to be imparted to a mixture of molecules to make them interact is appropriately known as the activation energy. Everyone is familiar with the sight of a Bunsen burner in an old-fashioned chemistry laboratory (nowadays they use electric heaters instead); its purpose was to supply the activation energy to whatever reaction was under study. But there are other ways of getting molecules to bump into each other. Take the reaction between hydrogen and oxygen to form water:

$$2H_2 \ + \ O_2 \longrightarrow 2H_2O \ + \ energy$$
(hydrogen) (oxygen) (water)

This is potentially a highly explosive reaction, but only in the presence of a spark or other form of heat. At a low enough temperature, no reaction will occur. It can, however, be speeded up, in a more controlled manner, by adsorbing the gaseous hydrogen and oxygen onto the surface of a solid material such as palladium black (a form of the metal palladium). This, in effect, brings the molecules so close together that they react without the need for heat. The presence of the palladium black, which itself is unchanged by the reaction, has in effect lowered the activation energy to the point that reaction occurs at a much lower temperature than it otherwise would. Palladium black functions as a catalyst. Catalysts, then, lower the activation energy of chemical reactions, speeding up the rate at which those reactions take place. Let us return to the boy on his toboggan on top of the snow-covered hill. If he simply sits on his toboggan, it may not move, especially if the snow is wet. But if his friend comes along and gives him a slight push, he will start on his downward journey. The potential energy released by tobogganing from the top of the hill to the bottom is the same, irrespective of whether his friend has given him a push or not. What his friend has done is to supply the energy necessary to get him going: This is what activation energy is. Enzymes, which are one class of proteins, are no more than catalysts of biological origin. Every cell in our body, every cell in a tomato, contains enzymes.

Enzymes are very sophisticated catalysts indeed. They are so sophisticated that even many years after Wöhler's experiment of turning an inorganic salt into an organic molecule, scientists still argued about a "vital" force being responsible for biological catalysis. (Most of them were studying the fermentation of sugar to alcohol by extracts of yeast—never mind the complex reactions that occur in the human body!) It was the fact that enzymes like urease (splitting urea into ammonia and carbon dioxide) and pepsin (breaking down proteins in the stomach) could be made to form crystals—just like ordinary molecules—that finally knocked vitalism on its head. Enzymes are extremely specific, in contrast to palladium black, which catalyzes reactions because it has the capacity to adsorb gaseous molecules, and therefore catalyzes all kinds of reaction indiscriminately. Each step in the oxidation of glucose to carbon dioxide and water, which in the body is separated into more than 20 different reactions, is catalyzed by a separate enzyme. There are tens of thousands of different enzymes, each catalyzing a different reaction, in our bodies. While the basic reactions of energy utilization and of synthesis of carbohydrates, fats, proteins, DNA, and RNA are the same in all cells, it is the formation of specific molecules, such as actin and myosin in muscle and heart, urea and bile acids in liver, insulin in pancreas, neurotransmitters in brain, and so forth, that gives each organ its individual function; the synthesis of every different molecule requires the presence of one or more specific enzymes. The basic energy-utilizing and synthetic reactions are common to all animals and plants. But the synthesis of the green pigment of plants (chlorophyll) that is involved in the capture of light energy to form carbohydrate, requires different reactions and hence different enzymes than those required to form the skin of reptiles or the hide of elephants; the formation of pink-pigmented orchids requires different enzymes than the formation of violet-pigmented orchids, and blue-eyed people require different enzymes for the formation of retinal pigment than do brown-eyed people. In short, the differences between the various tissues within one organism, and the differences between the myriad of plants and animals on the globe, are related to the fact that each tissue and each organism contains a slightly different set of enzymes. And each different enzyme, i.e., each different protein, is specified by a different gene. It is through enzymes that the genetic diversity of all living matter is expressed.

Exactly how do enzymes work? Part of the mechanism is the same as that by which palladium black catalyzes the reaction between hydrogen and oxygen: by bringing the necessary molecules closer together. Enzymes therefore have specific binding sites for each of the participating molecules in a particular reaction. It is by binding only 1 of 1000 different molecules that the specificity of enzymes is realized (see Figure 61 in Chapter 7 for a computer graphic image of this). A combination lock has thousands of possible numbers for unlocking it, but only one actually works. So it is with enzymes. But enzymes do more than just bind other molecules. They facilitate the course of a reaction by actually participating in it: by making and breaking covalent bonds between the reacting molecules and some of the amino acids of which the enzyme is composed. Just as the oxidation of glucose to carbon dioxide and water is split up into more than 20 separate reactions in living organisms, so any one reaction catalyzed by an enzyme (as all reactions in living matter are) is split into many steps. But these are not discrete stages like the 20 reactions into which glucose oxidation is split. Rather the enzyme and the reacting molecules undergo continuous and subtle changes of structure so that no single step involves a large energy difference. The changes are more akin to the contortions of a circus performer or a ballet dancer. Of course the enzyme (like the dancer) finishes up in its original form at the end of the reaction, otherwise it would not be a catalyst so much as another reactant molecule. Another analogy is an automated production line. At each stage a machine takes two parts, puts them together, passes them on, and is then ready to accept two further parts and to repeat the process; the machine is the catalyst for putting the two parts together. In older times it was a human being who was the catalyst, though there are still examples enough of human beings working in this way. Just as human beings, and machines, wear out with time and need to be replaced, so do enzymes. Enzymes, in contrast to long-lived proteins like those of muscle, connective tissue, or nerve, have relatively short lifetimes: days, or even hours, as opposed to months or years. That is to say, they are being continuously broken down (by other enzymes) and resynthesized (by reading off the appropriate gene, which also involves other enzymes).

The ability of enzymes to recognize specific molecules and then to transform them into other molecules requires a very specific structure, as well as a flexibility to undergo the subtle changes mentioned above. Both are provided by enzymes being proteins. For proteins are the most varied molecules known. Of the 100,000 or so different proteins in a human being, no two are exactly alike. Given that there are over 2 million different species of animals and plants today (over 15 million species have become extinct), there must be billions of different proteins in existence.

Yet each protein consists of the same 20 amino acids strung together—in different sequences—along a linear strand. Our perplexity as to how so many different structures can be formed from a mere 20 different units is quickly dispelled by a mathematician. He will immediately tell us that if an average protein contains some 100 amino acids, which is a reasonable figure, there are 20^{100} different ways of assembling them; and 20^{10}— never mind 20^{100}—is already 10 billion. So, no problem. Actually many potential combinations of amino acids are never found; there are virtually no proteins that have runs of more than 6 of the same amino acid in a row, whereas the figure of 20^{100} of course includes proteins made up entirely of a single amino acid. Also, most animal proteins have all 20 amino acids in them (some plant proteins have only 18 or 19, which can lead to nutritional deficiencies in strict vegetarians), which is another restriction. The point of this argument is to emphasize how much variability can be achieved from just 20 different units assembled in rows of some 100 units long. The way this information is stored and passed from generation to generation in genes is even more economical: just 4 different nucleotides (A, G, C, and T), read off in groups of 3 (which provides 64 different combinations—4^3 being 64—and therefore more than enough to code for 20 different amino acids). This economy of structural units—just 4 nucleotides and 20 amino acids to code for, and to comprise, over 10 billion different proteins—has been shared by plants and animals for over a billion years, and by the earliest microbes for 3 billion years before that. How did it all evolve? Were there originally fewer amino acids, which were then found wanting, or more, which were then found redundant? And how were the actual structures of the nucleotides and amino acids selected from the billions of possible combinations of C, H, O, N, P, and S? It is for these reasons that it would be fascinating if organic molecules were found on another planet—and Mars seems the only likely candidate (though Europa, one of the moons of Jupiter, is another possibility because it contains water)—and brought back for chemical analysis. Comparison of Martian molecules with those on Earth would provide remarkable insight as to how molecular evolution works.

This digression was prompted by a consideration of protein structure in relation to enzymatic activity. How is a protein folded so as to create highly specific sites—generally some form of indentation or pocket—into which particular molecules can fit, and how does the structure of an enzyme change during the catalytic act? The first question is especially important, since binding of particular molecules to specific sites on proteins is the basis not only of enzymatic catalysis but of many other biological processes that involve the binding of particular molecules to proteins. The action of hormones is one. A hormone is a molecule that is produced in one tissue and acts to control metabolism in other tissues; it is carried around the bloodstream—the word is derived from the Greek "to carry"—until it meets the appropriate receptor protein, often on the surface of the cell it is programmed to influence. Immune mechanisms, transmission of nerve impulses, gene recognition, and a host of other processes, some of which will be described in the chapters that follow, are other examples. It is no exaggeration to say that virtually all molecular events that occur in cells result from the binding of a particular molecule to a specific site on a protein. The way that a protein folds so as to expose some of its amino acids and to bury others within it is dictated by the sequence of amino acids that make up the protein. As the protein is synthesized it begins to fold; bonds are formed between different parts of the protein in such a way that the form that is finally adopted is that of lowest energy. What are these bonds?

First there are covalent bonds between the S atom of one cysteine residue (cysteine is an amino acid that contains sulfur) and the S atom of another cysteine residue. These are generally quite far apart in the linear sequence of amino acids; it is the bonding that brings them together and results in the folding of the protein. Then there are hydrogen (H) bonds between particular oxygen and nitrogen atoms, as described earlier. There are also ionic interactions between some positively charged and some negatively charged amino acids, generally on the surface of a protein. Finally there are interactions between the fatlike, hydrophobic (water-hating, hence water-avoiding) regions of different amino acids; roughly half of the 20 different amino acids have hydrophobic

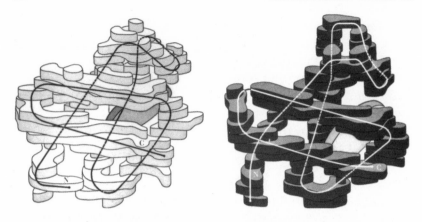

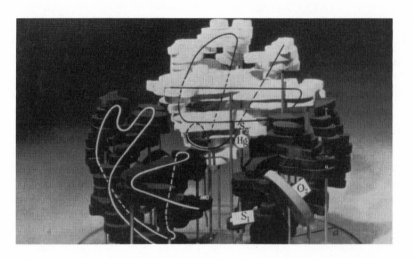

19. Hemoglobin. Hemoglobin is a typical globular, water-soluble protein. The molecule is made up of four separate molecules or amino acid chains, held together: there are two A or α chains and two B or β chains, which differ slightly from each other. The top picture shows an α chain (consisting of 141 amino acids) in white and a β chain (consisting of 146 amino acids) in black. The small blocks that resemble jigsaw pieces, are "election density" maps—based on X-ray diffraction analysis of crystals of α and β chains—which indicate the positions of individual amino acids. The position of the heme group in each molecule is indicated by the flat circular disk, shown in darker shading for the α chain and in lighter shading for the β chain. The continuous line (black for the α chain and white for the β chain) indicates the sequence in which the amino acids are joined together. The compact, folded structure of each molecule results regions created by $CH_3CH_2CH_2-$ and similar residues. Recall the discussion of phospholipids: Through their avoidance of water, fatlike, hydrophobic portions of one molecule develop a mutual attraction for the fatlike portion of another molecule, just as in a group of children the weaker—often brighter—ones avoid the stronger—often more sportive—ones, and form relationships among themselves through the avoidance of the other group. In the case of proteins, the hydrophobic regions are not on separate molecules, but within the same molecule.

The net result of all of these bondings is that proteins finish up in a compact, globular structure (Figure 19), with most of their hydrophobic amino acids buried in the middle of the protein and most of the hydrophilic (water-loving) amino acids on the outside, where they make contact with water through H bonds. This, then, would be the structure of a typical protein such as an enzyme, as well as of hemoglobin. Other proteins that have a structural rather than an enzymatic role adopt quite different configurations. Examples are the actin and myosin fibers of muscle (Figure 69 in Chapter 8), the collagen fibers of connective tissue, and the keratin fibers of hair. Of all of the bonds that keep a protein in its folded state, H bonds are the most important (some proteins, for example, have no covalent S bonds). And having the correct shape is crucial for a protein if it is to function as an enzyme. Break H bonds, say by heating, and the ability of an enzyme to catalyze a molecular interaction is lost. Without enzymes there is no life, just as without DNA and RNA there is no life. The activity of all three molecules—proteins, DNA, and RNA—depends on H bonds. It is the relatively mild temperatures on the surface of the globe that has allowed life as we know it to evolve. Deeper in the earth's crust, in volcanos for example, there can be

---

from many hydrogen bonds formed between individual amino acids. The bottom picture shows how the α and the β chains interact in the full hemoglobin molecule; the two β chains (in black) and one of the α chains (in white) are indicated. The position at which oxygen (O_2) binds to the heme group in a cavity created by folding of the right-hand β chain is shown. Photographs by courtesy of Dr. Max Perutz, MRC Laboratory of Molecular Biology, Cambridge, from models built by him in 1959.

no life because the temperature, as a result of residual radioactive explosions, is thousands of degrees too high for any H bonds to survive.

———————————◆◄———————

Molecules, then, are extremely small. A molecule of water, which is the most abundant molecule in all living things, is a million times smaller than the point of a very fine needle. Even the largest molecule of life—DNA—cannot be seen with the naked eye. Between these two extremes are molecules like glucose, fatty acids, and amino acids that are some 10 times larger than water, and proteins that are some 1000 times larger. These molecules are present in every part of our body. The way they interact with each other underlies every one of our body functions. But we are not unique: The same molecules, the same interactions, occur in every animal, in every plant, in every microbe. In the chapters that follow we shall see how these molecules of life participate in our own bodies in health and disease.

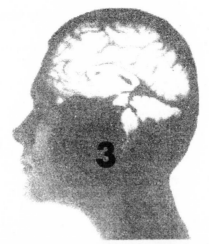

THE HEALTHY BODY

NUTRITION AND METABOLISM

The position of the major organs in the body is shown in Figure 20. The heart plays a central role, which is to push blood to all tissues and organs of the body. This function is preeminent because the blood brings to every cell, in every tissue and organ, the nutrients it needs to remain alive. These nutrients are primarily oxygen and glucose. The oxygen is picked up from the lungs, which it enters via the windpipe or trachea every time one takes a breath. There is a separate circulation from heart to lungs and back to the heart (Figure 21). Oxygenated blood is then pumped throughout the rest of the body; this is known as the arterial system. Oxygen-depleted blood is returned back to the heart and on to the lungs; this is known as the venous system. Glucose and other nutrients derived from the food that we eat are absorbed from the intestines and enter the arterial system. After passing through the liver and the other organs and tissues of the body, venous blood return to the heart and hence to the lungs depleted of oxygen, and enriched in carbon dioxide. On reaching the lungs, carbon dioxide, which eventually appears in

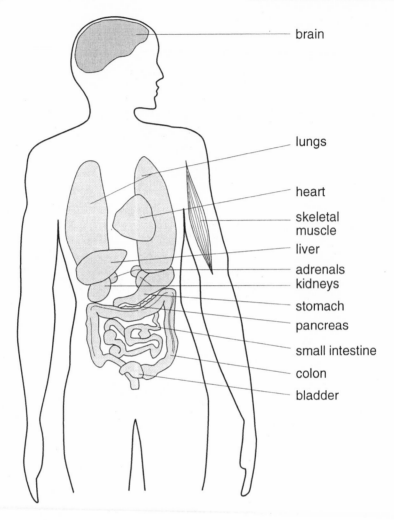

20. Tissues and organs of the body. From *An Introduction to Human Biochemistry* by C. A. Pasternak, Oxford University Press, 1979.

the exhaled breath, is exchanged for oxygen, and the whole cycle is repeated.

Breathing is accelerated when we become extremely anxious, as a result of a process known as hyperventilation. This is one reason why motorists who are caught in a snowdrift, and

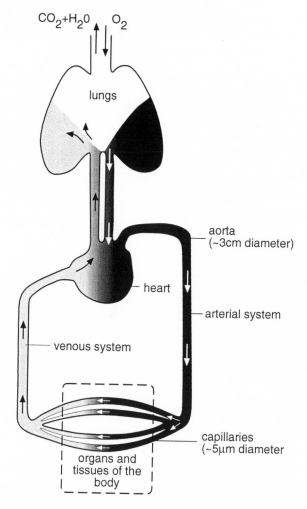

CO_2+H_2O O_2

lungs

aorta
(~3cm diameter)

heart

arterial system

venous system

capillaries
(~5µm diameter

organs and
tissues of the
body

21. Circulation of blood. The arrows indicate the direction of flow. The intensity of shading indicates the amount of oxygen in the blood. From *An Introduction to Human Biochemistry* by C. A. Pasternak, Oxford University Press, 1979.

close the windows of their car to retain heat, run out of oxygen faster than they otherwise would, and therefore die sooner. The same is true of children who place a plastic bag over their heads. In each case, the main reason is lack of oxygen, as discussed in

Chapter 2. The reason why people who put their heads in gas ovens die relatively quickly is different. It is because carbon monoxide in the gas mixture binds hemoglobin in the blood more tightly than oxygen; indeed any bound oxygen is displaced by carbon monoxide. Insufficient oxygen therefore reaches the cells of organs like heart and brain, and death ensues. For this and other reasons, modern commercial gas contains methane in place of carbon monoxide. Scientists have recently found that carbon monoxide—at very low concentration—may play a role in long-term memory, but people of a forgetful nature are not encouraged to try inhaling carbon monoxide to improve their retention: They are likely to end up in the Big Sleep (as Raymond Chandler, author of the Philip Marlowe detective stories, put it), with no benefit to long-term memory.

Just how much work does the heart have to do? The total volume of blood in an average person is some 5.5 liters (approximately 12 pints). Almost the entire amount circulates through the heart every minute. This requires an enormous amount of energy, because the heart is pumping blood against a very high resistance. What is the nature of this resistance? It is that the arteries, through which blood leaves the heart, divide into progressively more, and progressively smaller, vessels (arterioles and capillaries) that deliver oxygen and the other nutrients of blood to all tissues of the body. Eventually the capillaries unite with other capillaries to form progressively larger vessels until blood (depleted of oxygen but enriched in carbon dioxide) finally reenters the heart through the veins. Although an average capillary is no more than 1 mm (1/25th of an inch) in length, there are so many of them that their total length in body has been estimated to be near 25,000 miles. But it is their narrowness that creates the high resistance: about 5 μm (1/5000th of an inch) in width, just enough for a red blood cell to squeeze through. The heart must therefore exert a high pressure to force the blood through the body: between 75 and 125 mm of mercury, depending on which stage of the heartbeat the measurement is taken. Given that a healthy, resting heart is beating at around 72 beats/min, the heart in a resting individual probably uses more energy than any other organ.

The heartbeat, which can often be felt simply by putting one's hand over the chest, is generally measured as the pulse rate at some peripheral site like the arteries in the wrist. More accurate determinations of the timing of openings and closings of the heart are carried out with electrodes placed on the skin over the heart—the electrocardiograph (ECG); this is not to be confused with the electroencephalograph (EEG), which measures rhythmic fluctuations in the brain. In general, the more regularly the heart beats, the better; some irregularities—arrhythmias—are a sign of impending danger and can lead to death. However, *very* tiny irregularities in heartbeat are now known to be normal; indeed, a *completely* regular heart is often a sign of disease to come. How irregular should these small irregularities be? Recent work from Harvard University and Massachusetts Institute of Technology (MIT) has been investigating this problem. The answer appears to be that the irregularities should not be completely random, but should rather follow chaos theory, i.e., be chaotic. What is this theory? First it should be noted that the words chaos and chaotic are particularly ill-chosen and misleading, since they refer to events that are *not* totally random. Chaos theory states that some seemingly random events are not, in fact, random when analyzed in a particular way. Instead, they have an element of predictability about them, because any chaotic event that occurs is dependent on what has preceded it. Nonchaotic events lack this dependency. Chaotic events abound before our eyes. The rise and fall of the waves in the ocean may appear to be random, but is in fact dependent on previous events: As the surfers of southern California know, the ninth wave is usually the big one. The way in which the currents created by El Niño in the southern Pacific eventually cause floods in one part of the world and droughts in another, is chaotic. The fall of a particular leaf off a tree in autumn is chaotic because it is dependent on previous interactions between leaf and stalk. At the molecular level, the movement of nitrogen molecules in air is indeed random, but when a protein molecule is being made, the strands of its constituent amino acids fold up in a chaotic manner as they grow longer and longer. The movement of ions like Na^+ and K^+ through the narrow channels across the membrane of our nerve cells may also be chaotic rather than random.

What the researchers at Harvard and MIT did was to measure the heartbeat of patients with an ECG during the night, while the person was asleep and the overall heartbeat therefore stable. By recording the data on a small computer, the scientists confirmed that the heartbeat of a healthy person displays tiny irregularities: These were shown by mathematical analysis to be chaotic, not random. The supposition is that lack of irregularities, or random rather than chaotic ones, signals danger. The software for this kind of analysis is now being developed for home use so that one will be able to check one's heart while asleep. Should the recordings show an absence of chaotic irregularities, one could then seek medical treatment. However, most of us will worry so much about what our heart is, or is not, doing in the middle of the night, that we are likely to lose a lot of sleep and to develop the symptoms of stress, which is in itself a powerful stimulus for heart disease. Moreover, some people can take bad news well, others not. We may indeed be at the point where frequent or continual monitoring of what the molecules in our body are doing is beneficial; but for many, that knowledge is likely to be counterproductive.

We have seen that, next to oxygen, water is the most crucial molecule needed for life to occur. Life developed in a watery environment, and all of the molecular interactions that have made life possible ever since have been taking place in a watery solution. Actually the solution is quite strong in salt: around 0.9% salt in all of the cells and fluids of the human body, which is almost a third as strong as seawater. Indeed, lack of salt in the diet is almost as serious as lack of water. Why, it may be asked, are water and salt so crucial? Neither is used up in energy-yielding reactions. On the contrary, water is *produced* during the oxidation of carbohydrate and other nutrients, as was seen in the last chapter. If the circulation is indeed a closed system like a central heating system, why should water and salt need to be replaced? The answer is that the circulation is not a perfectly sealed system, and there is a continual drainage of water and salt out of it. This happens in the kidneys.

The first part of the kidneys is a filter (the glomerulus) designed to allow water and small molecules like glucose and waste products like urea, the nitrogen-containing molecule that is the end product of protein breakdown, to pass through. Large molecules like protein are retained. So of course are the red and white blood cells and the cell fragments called thrombocytes or platelets that are involved in blood clotting. A fairly common disease, generally the end result of an infection elsewhere in the body or the ingestion of a toxic substance that becomes concentrated in the kidney, is glomerulonephritis: The condition refers to damage to the nephron at the filtration stage. A nephron (Figure 22) is a narrow tube or tubule that collects the watery filtrate in the glomerulus at its top end. The nephron then becomes highly convoluted and eventually joins with all of the other nephrons in the kidney to pass their contents into the bladder; from there the fluid is eventually excreted as urine. In glomerulonephritis, the filter of the glomerulus becomes damaged and leaky, so that protein appears in the urine. Loss of protein is deleterious because the proteins in blood perform important functions. The most abundant protein is albumin and one of its major roles is to prevent seepage of water into the tissues of the body, a condition known as edema. Other proteins are present in much smaller amounts. Although such proteins also perform important functions, they are not directly affected in glomerulonephritis. At this stage the reader should merely note three other classes of protein found in the bloodstream: hormones, which coordinate the various metabolic reactions that take place in different tissues of the body; enzymes responsible for blood clotting, which—together with platelets—prevents the loss of blood through damaged capillaries; and components of the immune system, which protects the body against infection.

In the second part of the kidney, in which the nephron becomes highly convoluted, 99% of the water and even more of the salt that has passed through the glomerular filter is reabsorbed into the bloodstream; of the organic molecules present, glucose is absorbed with 100% efficiency, but urea with only 40% efficiency. The result is that the urine that finally emerges is much enriched in urea and other waste products. (It is the slow breakdown of urea to ammonia—partially by bacteria such as *Proteus mirabilis* and partially nonenzymatically—that gives old lavatories—and

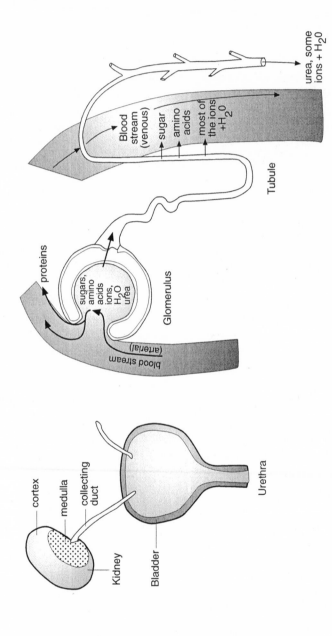

22. Role of kidneys. (a) Flow through one of the kidneys into the bladder. (b) A single nephron is shown. From *An Introduction to Human Biochemistry* by C. A. Pasternak, Oxford University Press, 1979.

cow sheds—their distinct odor.) The retention in urine of only 1% of the water that was present in blood does not seem like very much, but it has to be remembered that some 180 liters (47 gallons) of water passes through the kidney per day, giving rise to 1.5 to 1.8 liters (3 to 4 pints) of urine. By the same token, the amount of salt that passes through the kidney is 1.5 kg (3.3 lb) per day. The reabsorption from nephron to blood of large amounts of water, salt, and glucose requires a large amount of energy; over 90% of the energy obtained by the kidney from the breakdown of nutrients is devoted to the reabsorption process. Kidney failure—which affects some 3 million people in the United States, 25,000–75,000 of whom die of the disease annually—generally leads to an *increase* in salt and water, as well as toxic waste products, in the blood. This is because it is generally filtration through the glomerulus, not reabsorption from the nephron, that fails. As a result, water is retained in tissues, the condition previously referred to as edema, and they swell. Swollen ankles and other limbs are a typical feature of kidney failure. The cause of the renal failure, which leads to such edema, is often an infection, the ingestion of a toxic substance, a tumor, or a kidney stone. The most common cause of edema, however, is a failing heart (congestive heart failure). A lot of pressure has to be exerted to push the blood through the body, and a fall in cardiac output due to a weak heart leads directly to edema. It is not surprising, therefore, that some of the most frequently prescribed drugs are diuretics (increasing the output of urine). Different classes of these drugs act at different sites, but the end result is the same: a restored flow of urine. Actually the kidneys are able to compensate for minor failures in function fairly well—remember that one can survive on only one kidney—and it is only in extreme cases that disease ensues.

Water, then, is continuously being lost from the circulation by way of the kidneys. The underlying reason for such an apparently wasteful process is probably that it provides a pathway for excreting end products of metabolism and toxic substances that an individual may have unintentionally consumed. The kidney is not the only place where water is lost. An average person ingests about 2½ liters (more than 5 pints) of water per day. Half of this is ingested as fluids, the other half enters the body as food (recall that more than 60% of all living matter is water). 1½ liters (just over 3 pints), in other words 60%, is lost through the kidneys. Of the remaining 40%, most is lost through the lungs (we all know that if we breathe onto a cold surface like glass, water condenses on it), with the rest secreted as sweat and excreted in the feces. Of course this is for an average person, in an equable climate. In hot climates more water is lost as sweat, and this—together with the salt that accompanies it—needs to be replenished by drinking more water and eating salty foods. The two go together: Eating more salt makes one drink more. The body has sensors that try to keep the internal environment just right: for thirst, for appetite, and as described above, for breathing also. Of course there are situations where the control mechanisms are overpowered. One example is the severe diarrhea that is caused by infectious bacteria like cholera and pathogenic strains of *Escherichia coli*. By interacting with the normally absorptive cells of the small intestine they cause these to do the opposite: to secrete large amounts of water and salt—up to 15 liters a day. More than 3 million children a year were dying of this type of dehydration 20 years ago. Vaccination against cholera has not proved very effective. What has saved millions of lives in India and Bangladesh has been a trivially simple invention: a double-ended plastic spoon. In one cavity is placed glucose, in the other common salt (NaCl). The absorption of glucose in the small intestine is known to bring Na^+ with it, which then pulls Cl^- in (to preserve electrical neutrality), and most importantly, water (to maintain the concentrations of ions inside cells). Recall that this is also the mechanism for the absorption of water back into the bloodstream in the kidney (see Figure 22 above). By eating glucose and salt, and drinking boiled water, the loss of salt and water is largely overcome and the diarrhea halted, at least long enough for the patient to survive. It is as a result of this simple procedure that the death rate of children from cholera has fallen from 50–60% to less than 1%.

How is the intake of food controlled? There exists in the brain a sensor for appetite, as shown by the Russian scientist Ivan Pavlov (Figure 23) over 100 years ago. Pavlov trained dogs to salivate every time he rang a bell, having first rung a bell every

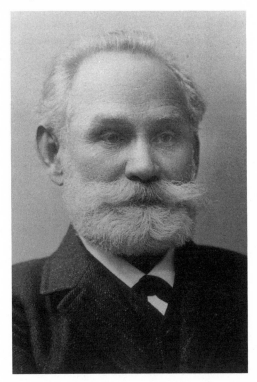

23. Ivan Pavlov. Nobel laureate, 1904. Copyright: The Nobel Foundation, Stockholm.

time food was given to the dogs. This was an important experiment, not only because it demonstrated an important physiological control mechanism, but because it showed that the mind and the rest of the body are closely connected. I shall return to this topic in Chapter 6. For now it should be noted that Pavlov's experiment was a perfectly humane one. What of other experiments with animals? This is a fairly hot area of debate for many people, so I will pause for a moment to discuss it.

It was experiments with dogs—all under anesthesia, though regrettably the dogs were put down in the end—that led to the first human heart transplant and subsequently to transplants of kidney and liver as well. Thousands of human lives have been saved as a result of these pioneering experiments. Equally unavoidable are the many animal experiments—generally with mice and rats—by which the toxicity of new drugs against heart disease, kidney failure, cancer, and every other disease amenable to therapeutic treatment has been assessed.

The use of human cells in culture to test the toxicity of novel drugs is an excellent tool that cuts down the number of animal experiments that need to be performed, but it is not sufficient. It cannot, for example, predict possible side effects in kidney, liver, brain, or lung. We should be thankful that the molecular basis of health and disease in other mammals is so similar to ours, and that we are not driven to using orphans or prisoners for testing potentially lifesaving drugs (as has been done by inhumane regimes in the past). This is not to say that one should condone some of the ridiculous experiments that have been carried out so as to assess—for example—the effects on body weight and state of mind of rats kept running on a treadmill by application of an electric shock every time they pause for breath (the result being the obvious and predictable one that rats lose weight and become mentally stressed). Fortunately, most countries now have pretty stringent animal welfare laws that forbid those kinds of experiments. In any case, there are enough experiments carried out on human volunteers like elite athletes who are only too anxious to know exactly what the relationship between exercise and body weight might be, and—as will be discussed in a subsequent chapter—there is a wealth of information now accumulating as to the many consequences of stress in humans, to make these kinds of experiments on animals unnecessary.

Having discussed the roles played by the heart, lungs, and kidneys, the function of the liver will now be considered (Figure 24). The liver has several roles. First, it processes the food that is absorbed through the intestines. Because this is such an important function, a special blood supply (the hepatic portal vein) brings the products of digestion directly from the intestines to the liver. Only after blood has perfused the liver is it passed to the heart. The main molecules that are absorbed from the intestines are sugars and amino acids; they are derived from the breakdown of carbohydrate and protein, respectively. The enzymes responsible for

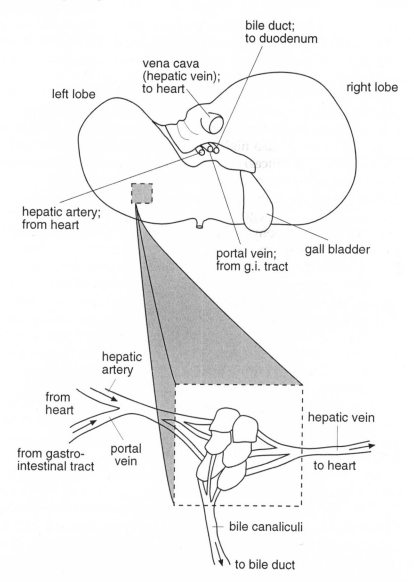

24. The liver. The upper drawing shows the organ in relation to incoming (from hepatic artery and portal vein) and outgoing (from hepatic vein) blood. The position of gallbladder and bile duct are indicated. The lower drawing shows a group of liver cells (hepatocytes) in relation to incoming and outgoing fluids. From *An Introduction to Biochemistry* by C. A. Pasternak, Oxford University Press, 1979.

the breakdown of carbohydrate are called amylases (starch is also known as amylose); the enzymes that break down protein are pepsin, chymotrypsin, and trypsin. Enzymes that break down triglyceride (a fat, or lipid) are known as lipases. The process of breakdown, that is, the digestion of food, takes place in the alimentary tract (Figure 25). Digestion occurs predominantly in the stomach and the small intestine; the latter organ is not only long (some 20 feet) but also highly convoluted into crypts (pockets) and villi (protuberances) so as to generate maximal surface area for optimal absorption. As mentioned in the preceding chapter, the main carbohydrate of animal food, especially of meat (i.e., muscle tissue), is glycogen, which is made up entirely of glucose units. The main carbohydrate of plant food is starch, which is also made up only of glucose. But two important sources of carbohydrate contain sugars other than glucose: Lactose of milk contains one unit of glucose and one of galactose, and sucrose (the only really sweet sugar) from sugarcane or sugar beet—presented in a thousand different ways by the confectionary industry—contains one unit of glucose and one of fructose. Both galactose and fructose, each of which has the same composition as glucose—namely, $C_6H_{12}O_6$—are turned into glucose by specific enzymes as, of course, are all of the other molecular changes that take place in the liver. The glucose is then passed to all other tissues for breakdown to CO_2 and H_2O or—in times of plenty—is retained in the liver for synthesis of glycogen. Protein, which is present in all animal foods and, to a lesser degree, in the roots and fruits of plants, is broken down to amino acids. It will be recalled that all amino acids contain nitrogen; this is removed by the liver to form urea [NH_2CONH_2; essentially two molecules of ammonia (NH_3) linked to one of CO_2], which is excreted through the kidneys. The rest of the amino acid, having lost its N atom, is converted either to glucose or to a group of small molecules (containing four carbon atoms) called ketone bodies. Thus, the products of the degradation of carbohydrate and protein are glucose and ketone bodies. Together they provide the main energy source for tissues like muscle, heart, and kidneys. The brain is more discriminating and uses glucose only, except during periods of starvation, when it adapts to using ketone bodies as well.

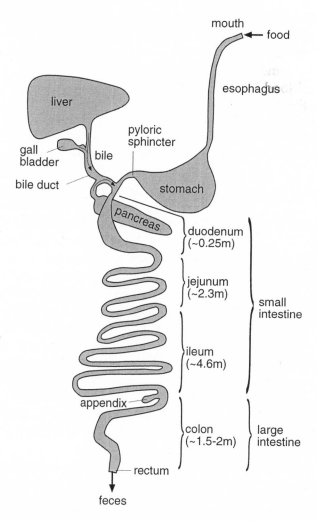

25. The alimentary tract. From *An Introduction to Human Biochemistry* by C. A. Pasternak, Oxford University Press, 1979.

So far we have not mentioned the breakdown and absorption of fat. Although it too occurs in the intestines, it is not absorbed through the hepatic portal vein, but through a special series of vessels and capillaries, known as the lymphatic system. This is a series of vessels, similar to blood vessels, that eventually empty into the bloodstream. Any fat that is broken down in the intestine is actually resynthesized to triglyceride in the absorptive cells before entering the lymphatics; cholesterol in the diet follows the same route. Both cholesterol and triglyceride circulate in the blood in the form of fat droplets or vesicles, as illustrated in Figure 13 in the previous chapter. Those that do not contain cholesterol are absorbed directly by the adipose (fat) cells. Here triglyceride is stored as an energy source for subsequent use. Those that do contain cholesterol are processed by the liver into somewhat smaller vesicles. The trouble with cholesterol is that once it is in the body, getting rid of it is extremely difficult. And on top of that, the liver itself synthesizes cholesterol. The reason why the body cannot rid itself of cholesterol is simple; it is one of a few molecules synthesized in the body that cannot be completely degraded by appropriate enzymes in particular tissues. Carbohydrate, triglyceride, protein, DNA, and RNA—all of which are synthesized in the body—can also all be broken down by it, eventually to CO_2 and H_2O.

Cholesterol is unique. To be sure, it is partially broken down to bile acids by the liver, but, as explained below, this is a very limited process. Cholesterol is also broken down, by oxidation of some of its carbon atoms, to other steroids. Steroids are molecules made up of four carbon rings as illustrated for cholesterol (itself a steroid) in Figure 10 in Chapter 2. These other steroids all function as hormones. Hormones, it will be recalled, are chemical messengers that circulate in the bloodstream. They are produced in one organ, and act to control metabolism in another organ. Most hormones either are proteins, like insulin, or are steroids, produced by partial breakdown of cholesterol. The main steroid hormones are cortisol, produced in the adrenals, and progesterone and the sex hormones (testosterone and estrogen) produced in testis and ovary. Because hormones act catalytically, like enzymes, they are present in the body in small amounts, and their formation from cholesterol accounts for only a minor part of its breakdown. Another minor breakdown product of cholesterol is vitamin D. This occurs when skin is exposed to the ultraviolet radiations of sunlight. Cholesterol itself is excreted, along with bile, into the duodenum, but some 50% is reabsorbed lower down the large intestine whence it reenters the circulation (Figure 26). Since cholesterol tends to be deposited along with other material in arteries, causing them to "furr" up and narrow, it is a major contributing factor to atherosclerosis or atheromatous disease. The process may be likened to the way a kettle "furrs" up with deposited calcium salts in regions of particularly hard, calcium-containing, water. In the case of arteries the deposit is a mixture of cholesterol, triglyceride, protein, and dead cells, known as an atheroma or atheromatous plaque. In this condition, narrowing of the arteries has reached such a stage that blood can barely pass,

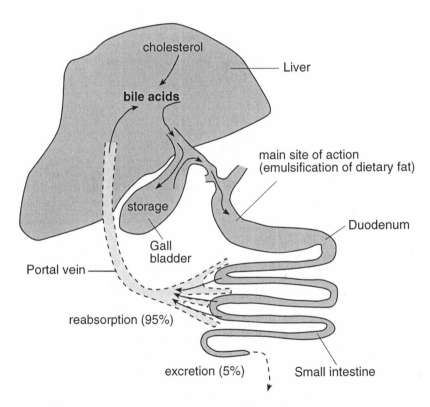

26. The circulation of bile. The values for reabsorption and excretion refer to bile acids. Cholesterol is approximately 50% reabsorbed and 50% excreted. From *An Introduction to Human Biochemistry* by C. A. Pasternak, Oxford University Press, 1979.

and there is danger of a complete block in circulation, brought on by the formation of a blood clot (as described below). If this happens in the arteries leading to the brain, the result is a stroke. If it happens in the arteries leading to the heart cells, which is an especially frequent outcome, the result is heart failure or coronary heart disease. It must be remembered that it is the individual heart cells, through their muscle filaments (see Figure 69 in Chapter 8)—made up of actin, myosin, and other proteins all working in unison—that cause the heart to beat. These cells are critically dependent on a supply of oxygen and nutrients like glucose, fatty acids, or ketone bodies (an alternative, four-carbon-atom, energy source derived from protein or fat).

When that supply is blocked, a dangerous situation occurs. One way to ameliorate matters is to try to dissolve the offending plaque away with enzymes, and a major goal of the pharmaceutical industry is the synthesis of appropriate human enzymes (so as to prevent an immune response) to do just this. Another technique is to insert a short tube, called a stent, that is coated with biocompatible material in order to prevent further deposits. Alternatively the artery may be expanded by introducing a balloon on the end of a catheter and then inflating the balloon, a technique known as angioplasty. Another procedure is a bypass operation, the faulty artery literally being bypassed through the insertion of an alternative vessel. But by far the best way is to try to prevent the situation from ever occurring by limiting the intake of cholesterol and other fat. Unfortunately the situation is not as simple as this, as cholesterol is not the only precipitating factor. In fact there is currently very little evidence that lowering blood cholesterol has any effect on preventing atherosclerosis in people who have not already suffered a heart attack. It is only in those who have, that lowering blood cholesterol appears to be beneficial. Indeed it may be noted that as many as 40% of men who have a heart attack do so without being in any of the high-risk groups: no atherosclerosis, no high-fat diet, no high blood pressure, no lack of exercise, no smoking, no stress. We still have much to learn about the causes of heart disease! In the meantime we have to focus on those risk factors that we do know about. There are essentially two ways of lowering blood cholesterol: the first is to limit the intake of foods like eggs and cream that contain it; the second is to prevent the liver from synthesizing it. There is, in fact, a molecular "feedback" that does this anyhow: If the circulating cholesterol level is too high, it switches off cholesterol synthesis in the liver. The mechanism by which this happens is fairly complicated; it was worked out by two American scientists—Michael Brown and Joseph Goldstein (Figure 27), who received a Nobel Prize for their efforts. However, in some people one of the proteins involved in this process is missing. This is the result of the absence of the relevant gene: At an incidence of 0.2% of live births, it is one of the most common inherited disorders. Such people suffer from particularly high levels of cholesterol in the blood, known as cholesterolemia. Fortunately there are now several drugs on the market—lovastatin is one such molecule—that directly inhibit cholesterol synthesis. Other drugs—cholestyramine is one—prevent the reabsorption of bile from the intestine and therefore remove cholesterol from the circulation.

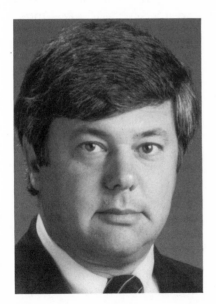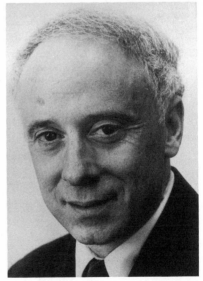

27. Michael Brown (left) and Joseph Goldstein. Nobel laureates, 1985. Copyright: The Nobel Foundation, Stockholm.

One of the functions of the liver, then, is to process the nutrients absorbed from the intestine into molecules that can be used directly for energy and growth. Another is to synthesize molecules required for a variety of different functions. The synthesis of cholesterol, from which several different hormones are derived, has already been mentioned; the formation of bile acids also starts with cholesterol. Bile is the brownish yellow, bitter fluid that we are familiar with when we vomit. Its main constituents are the bile acids. These are molecules that have both a water-soluble (hydrophilic) and a fat-soluble (hydrophobic) portion; they therefore resemble phospholipids (see the preceding chapter) and, like phospholipids, associate with each other to form micelles in which the water-soluble portions are on the outside making contact with water, while the fat-soluble portions are buried inside, making contact with each other (see Figure 13 on p. 31). The function of bile acids is to act as detergents: to make soluble—at least in part—dietary fat so that it can be broken down by the enzymes (lipases) in the intestine. For this purpose bile acids are passed by the liver into a storage organ—the gallbladder—from which they are secreted into the duodenum, as shown in Figure 25, when required. Bile also contains cholesterol; as mentioned earlier, only half of this is lost in the feces, the rest being reabsorbed back into the bloodstream (Figure 26). Bile acids are reabsorbed even more effectively—some 95%—so their synthesis in the liver is a relatively minor event. Occasionally the cholesterol in the gallbladder will crystallize to form gallstones. If these are small enough, they may simply pass into the duodenum and finish up in the feces. But if they are larger, and happen to block the passageway between gallbladder and duodenum (known as the bile duct), serious complications may ensue. These are related not only to a failure to digest fat properly—which is then lost in the feces—but to digest protein and carbohydrate also. The reason for this is that the enzymes that break down protein, carbohydrate, and fat are synthesized in the pancreas, from which they enter the duodenum via the bile duct (Figure 25). If this is blocked, the whole digestive system is at risk.

Once a large gallstone has formed, it is quite difficult to remove. Surgery, of course, is one answer. In the recently developed technique of keyhole surgery, only a very narrow incision is made and the surgeon manipulates his knife with the aid of a small telescope. This has made the removal of gallstones (and other operations) an outpatient procedure. Trying to break the stone into small pieces that can be passed out of the bile duct is another. Breaking the stones up with shock waves, similar to the use of sonication or high-frequency sound to remove crust off metallic and other surfaces, is sometimes successful. Trying to dissolve the stone with suitable chemicals has proved less successful.

The liver synthesizes many proteins that are secreted into the bloodstream. One of these is albumin, which makes up half of the proteins in plasma (plasma is blood without its red and white cells). The major function of albumin is, as we saw above, osmotic, that is, it retains water in the bloodstream that would otherwise seep into the tissues of the body. Another function of albumin is to carry fatty acids around the body. These are released from adipose (fat) cells when the triglyceride that is stored inside them is broken down. The stimulus for this to happen is the secretion of a hormone called epinephrine (adrenaline) from the adrenal gland. What causes the secretion of epinephrine in the first place? It is a message from the brain that is sent in response to a requirement for extra energy, like the sight of a bus that one is running to catch. Fatty acids, like triglyceride and cholesterol, are insoluble in water. Unlike triglyceride or cholesterol, they are carried in the bloodstream not in the form of vesicles or micelles, but bound to albumin in a fatty (hydrophobic) pocket designed for this purpose. Fat-soluble vitamins, like A, D, E, and K, are transported in similar fashion. When albumin containing fatty acids passes by skeletal muscle, the fatty acids are absorbed into the muscle cells and used for energy. Fatty acids are also used by heart, kidneys, and most other tissues with the exception of brain.

An important class of blood proteins synthesized by the liver are those concerned with blood clotting. The fact that the blood platelets form part of the plug that seals off damaged arteries has already been mentioned. Another part of the plug, or clot, is the protein fibrin. A meshwork of fibers made of fibrin (hence the name) and platelets form a sticky mass that blocks small tears or holes in blood vessels in the way that the drain from a kitchen sink occasionally becomes blocked with a mixture of vegetable peelings and the fat from meat. Fibrin is made by the liver and secreted as fibrinogen, a precursor protein that is soluble and so does not itself form a clot. A series of enzymes secreted from the liver, each acting on the next in a kind of cascade, is required to turn fibrinogen into fibrin; calcium ions also play a role. These are the clotting factors. Their importance is illustrated by the fact that if one such factor, for example factor VIII, is missing because of a faulty gene, the individual is likely to suffer loss of blood at the slightest bruise: this is the condition known as hemophilia, which will be discussed at greater length in the next chapter. It can be kept at bay by the injection of factor VIII isolated from spent blood, which has led to many men being infected with the HIV virus from contaminated blood; as will be explained in the following chapter, hemophilia rarely occurs in women. It may be noted that of hundreds of hemophiliacs in Japan who became infected with HIV during the 1980s through transfusion with infected blood, very few passed the virus to their wives, despite normal sexual relations: The danger of becoming infected with HIV is much greater through blood than through seminal fluid (the watery solution in which sperm is ejaculated). Nowadays factor VIII is made by genetically engineering the human gene into bacteria, which then make factor VIII in large amounts. This avoids the problems associated with the isolation of factor VIII from blood.

Just as failure to form a blood clot leads to problems, so does failure to remove a clot once formed. There is therefore another system of enzymes in the blood that has the abilty to dissolve a clot once it has served its purpose. Since the formation of unwarranted clots—provoked by the presence of an atheromatous plaque in an artery as described above—is a major cause of coronary heart disease, there is much effort in the pharmaceutical industry to find ways of boosting the clot-dissolving mechanism. At the same time, of course, scientists are searching for ways to prevent the formation of a clot in the first place. Somewhat surprisingly, it turns out that low doses of aspirin are quite effective. Men without a history of heart disease who take one tablet of aspirin per day over several years appear to have a 50% reduction in incidence of heart attacks. The figure for women is probably similar, but it should be remembered that for some people, aspirin does cause side effects like stomach problems. Currently the manufacture of a protein involved in solubilizing clots from the relevant human gene and its administration to patients is proving hopeful: The protein is called tissue plasminogen activator or TPA for short. A microbial protein that dissolves clots, namely, the enzyme streptokinase, is under equally active investigation (as well as immensely costly legal battles with regard to patent rights).

The final function of the liver to be considered here is the synthesis of enzymes that help to rid the body of toxic breakdown products of food and ingested drugs. The synthesis of urea from amino acid breakdown and its excretion in urine has already been mentioned. If urea is not synthesized, ammonia builds up and this is toxic in high concentration. Another molecule present in body fluids that is detoxified in the liver is heme. Heme is an organic molecule containing iron that is linked to the protein globin to form hemoglobin; hemoglobin binds oxygen (on its iron atom) and carries it from the lungs to all of the other tissues of the body. The red blood cells, in which hemoglobin resides, have a finite life span of some 120 days. This means that 100 billion red cells are synthesized every day, at the end of which they are broken down by the spleen. The spleen contains cells that somehow recognize the molecular features of "aged" red cells. The hemoglobin that is released dissociates into heme and globin. The heme molecule loses its iron, which is recycled for the synthesis of fresh hemoglobin; the rest of the molecule is then partially degraded, in the liver, to form bilirubin. This molecule is made more water-soluble by joining to glucuronic acid. By virtue of its solubility, bilirubin glucuronide can be excreted via the bile. Unlike bile acids or cholesterol, bilirubin glucuronide is not reabsorbed in the lower intestine and is eliminated in the feces. Many potentially toxic substances are ingested, either involuntarily in food, or on purpose. The liver has special sets of enzymes that partially degrade such molecules and then link them to glucuronic acid so as to make them more water-soluble. Most are then excreted by the kidneys; secretion via the bile in the case of bilirubin is an exception. Heme is an example of a molecule present in food (red meat contains much hemoglobin) that is rendered more water-soluble by the detoxifying enzymes of the liver; phenobarbitone is an example of a drug taken deliberately.

From the foregoing discussion it is clear that the liver is an extremely important organ in terms of the many molecular rearrangements it is able to catalyze. Thus, liver failure, through an infection, excess alcohol consumption, and other causes, is a severe condition. One of the warning signs is often a yellow coloration to the skin (jaundice). One reason is that damaged liver cells are not able to detoxify heme properly, and bilirubin and its precursor products, which are yellow, accumulate. Excess heme related to breakdown of red cells, a condition known as hemolysis, also causes jaundice. Another reason for jaundice is a blocked bile duct; if this is blocked by a gallstone, bilirubin accumulates in the liver (as well, of course, as cholesterol and bile acids).

We turn now to a brief discussion of how oxidizing the molecules produced by the digestion and metabolism of food, namely, glucose, ketone bodies, and fatty acids, enables us to do work. How is the process of oxidation coupled to muscle contraction so that the boy who was tobogganing down the slope in the previous chapter is able to pull his sled up the hill once more? The details have been worked out during the past 70 years by physiologists and biochemists, many of whom have devoted their lives to this problem (Figure 28).

First it must be stressed that the pathways by which glucose, ketone bodies, and fatty acids are oxidized converge at a common point. It is at the final stages of oxidation, to carbon dioxide and water, from that point on that most of the energy is released. What type of molecule captures this energy and transfers it to muscle fibers so that we can move our limbs, maintain the beating of our heart, and cause our intestines to writhe so that the food inside them is pushed along as it is being digested? What

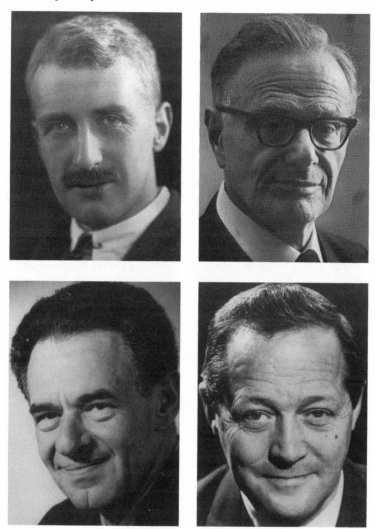

28. Archibald Hill, Hans Krebs, Fritz Lipmann, and Feodor Lynen. Top left: Hill (Nobel laureate, 1922) worked out the physiology of muscle contraction; Top right: Krebs (Nobel laureate, 1953) showed that pyruvic acid, an intermediate in the breakdown of glucose, is oxidized to carbon dioxide and water through a cyclic series of reactions; Bottom left: Lipmann (Nobel laureate, 1953) identified a key component in that cycle (coenzyme A, derived from the B vitamin pantothenic acid); Bottom right: Lynen (Nobel laureate, 1964) showed how fatty acids are oxidized to carbon dioxide and water (also involving coenzyme A). Copyright (Hill, Lipman, and Lynen): The Nobel Foundation, Stockholm.

type of molecule transfers energy to the walls of the kidney tubules so that 180 liters (47 gallons) of water, 1.5 kg (3.3 lb) of salt, and 0.2 kg (nearly half a pound) of glucose can be pushed through every day? What type of molecule transfers energy so that 100 billion red blood cells (plus numerous other cells) can be synthesized every day? It turns out to be the same molecule in all three cases, and indeed for every other energy-requiring reaction in the body. The molecule is ATP (adenosine triphosphate, a nucleotide like the building blocks of DNA and RNA, except that it has three phosphate groups, not one (see Figure 29). It is ATP that enables all of these processes to occur in tigers and elephants; it enables birds to fly halfway around the world, pythons to crush a dog in their coils, earthworms to wriggle, fireflies to glow, torpedo fish to stun their prey with an electric discharge strong enough to fell a man; that enables grass and wheat, orchids and giant sequoias to grow; and that enables salmonella and cholera, typhus and malaria, to invade us and multiply. In short, ATP has evolved as the common energy currency of every living thing.

How, then, is ATP formed and how does it provide energy to all of the processes mentioned above? The answer turns out to be

29. ATP. Structure of ATP [adenosine triphosphate; adenine (A) linked to ribose linked to three phosphate residues]. The arrow shows where ATP is split to form ADP (adenosine diphosphate; two phosphate residues). Note that AMP (adenosine monophosphate; one phosphate residue) is a building block of DNA and RNA. ATP, ADP, and AMP are nucleotides.

quite unexpected. For years biochemists had been searching for an organic compound that was formed during the oxidation of glucose, ketone bodies, and fatty acids that was somehow coupled to the synthesis of ATP. It was realized that the energy lies in the phosphate groups of ATP: that hydrolysis by water, to break the bond between two of the phosphate groups, releases more than three times as much energy as do other types of hydrolysis, such as that of breaking glycogen down to molecules of glucose, breaking triglycerides down to glycerol and fatty acids, or breaking proteins down to amino acids:

$$ATP + H_2O \longrightarrow ADP + phosphate + much\ energy$$

But to what type of "high-energy" molecule was phosphate—or ADP—linked in order to reverse the reaction and produce ATP? The answer, when it came, was so surprising that no one believed it. (This, of course, is fairly usual; scientists are born skeptics, which is why they always take so infuriatingly objective a view; just ask their spouses.) The situation was even worse because the man who came up with the answer was not the acknowledged leader of a great team, working in the latest, well-equipped laboratory and spending the taxpayer's money as if it were water. He was an eccentric Englishman, working with a few colleagues in the depths of the country, in an old farmhouse that he had converted with his own money into a small laboratory. His name was Peter Mitchell (Figure 30) and he sadly died a few years ago at age 71, in the Cornish farmhouse he had converted. The reason for the skepticism of the other contenders in the field was that the synthesis of ATP turned out not to involve an organic molecule at all!

It was known that glucose, fatty acids, and ketone bodies are oxidized to carbon dioxide and water inside small organelles called mitochondria (Greek for "threadlike structures"), which are present inside every cell of the body (except red blood cells). During the oxidation, hydrogen ions are transported from the mitochondria into the fluid in the rest of the cell (called cytoplasm). This pumping out of positively charged ions causes the membrane of mitochondria to become polarized, so that an electrical potential builds up across the mitochondrial membrane. Because

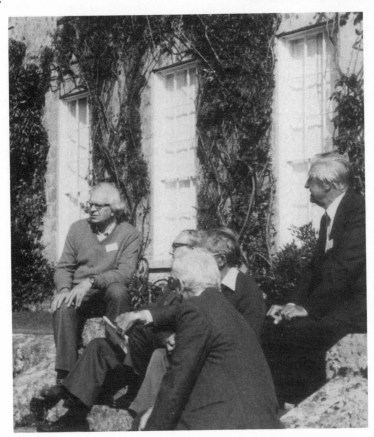

30. Peter Mitchell. Mitchell (Nobel laureate, 1978) is shown sitting on the extreme left, with a group of colleagues outside Glynn House in Bodmin, Cornwall. The occasion was a symposium in 1990 to mark the silver jubilee of Mitchell's conversion of part of the old house into laboratories in 1965.

positive charge is pumped out, the electrical potential across the mitochondrial membrane is negative inside, positive outside. We shall return to the induction of such potentials, called membrane potentials, in relation to nerve impulses in Chapter 8. The negative charge inside the mitochondrial membrane attracts hydrogen ions (H^+)—and any other positively charged ions like potassium (K^+) and calcium (Ca^{2+}) that are present in the cell's fluid—back into the mitochondria. But their membrane is not permeable to K^+

or Ca^{2+}. Nor, for that matter, is the membrane permeable to H^+, except through channels made of proteins that span the membrane and that are specifically permeable to H^+. On the inside of the membrane, i.e., within mitochondria, there are attached to the proteins that line the channel through which hydrogen ions flow, other proteins that are enzymes (Figure 31). These catalyze the following reaction:

$$ADP + phosphate + H^+ + much\ energy \longrightarrow ATP$$

The scientists searching for the energy-rich organic molecule had ignored the fact that the reverse reaction, the hydrolysis of ATP, releases a H^+. H^+ is an acid, but because all reactions inside

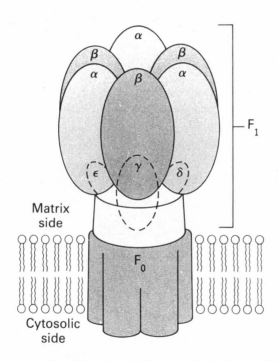

31. Proteins involved in ATP synthesis. The complex designated F_0 is the channel in the mitochondrial membrane through which hydrogen ions (H^+) are pulled. The complex, designated F_1, makes up the enzyme that synthesizes ATP from ADP, phosphate ion, and H^+ within mitochondria. From *Biochemistry* (4th edition) by L. Stryer, 1995. Used with permission of W. H. Freeman & Company.

cells take place in the presence of buffers that mop up any small amounts of acid or alkali (OH^-) produced, this did not seem to matter. In fact we now know that so strong is the electrical potential attracting positively charged ions into the mitochondrion that H^+ are attracted even out of a solution buffered at neutrality. But what is the source of the energy required to make ATP? Nothing more than the electrical potential across the mitochondrial membrane that is created by the oxidative processes occurring inside the mitochondrion. At this point the very perceptive reader will draw attention to an apparent paradox. Plants do not carry out oxidative processes (except in the dark). On the contrary, they catalyze the opposite reaction, namely,

$$6CO_2 \quad + \quad 6H_2O + energy \longrightarrow C_6H_{12}O_6 \quad + \quad 6O_2$$
(carbon dioxide) (water)   (carbohydrate) (oxygen)

Yet it was stated earlier that plants, too, use ATP as an energy-rich intermediate. What is going on? The answer is simple. The energy that drives the reaction of glucose synthesis and oxygen evolution is light energy, derived from the rays of the sun. Remember that the sun is undergoing nuclear explosions that release energy equivalent to the loss of 4 million tons of matter every second and that some of that energy, in the form of light, reaches us 9 minutes later. The chlorophyll that absorbs this energy is situated within chloroplasts, structures that are present in the cytoplasm (the watery fluid inside a plant cell) of all light-harvesting cells: shoots and leaves, but not roots or fruit. Chloroplasts are similar to mitochondria in structure and in function: They make ATP. Within chloroplasts, the absorption of light causes the expulsion of H^+ across the chloroplast membrane, creating an electrical potential—negative inside—just like in mitochondria. Again as in mitochondria, there is a specific H^+ channel, which is linked inside the chloroplast to an enzyme complex that synthesizes ATP (see Figure 31 on p. 83). Moreover, the H^+ channel protein and the ATP-synthesizing enzyme are remarkably similar in plants and animals. So here again, as in the structure of proteins, DNA, and RNA, there is a singularity of molecular structure that makes it difficult to escape from the idea that life as we know it evolved but once.

A healthy diet should contain protein, fat, and carbohydrate as well, of course, as water. Water does not mean wine or beer, even though these are more than 90% water. Moderate drinkers of wine, beer, or spirits should drink more water, not less, with their meals since alcohol is a diuretic, that is, it promotes the loss of water from the bloodstream through the kidneys. Water also flushes some of the toxic constituents of alcoholic drinks out of the system: A healthy intake of water to accompany alcoholic beverages prevents the headache and nausea of a hangover next day. Many studies of wine consumption—not surprisingly from countries like France and Italy—point to a beneficial effect of a glass or two of wine per day, and the same is true for beer. The reason is probably both nutritional and stress related. In these studies drinkers and nondrinkers were compared. The death rate among total abstainers was found to be higher than among moderate drinkers. But thereafter an increase in alcohol consumption correlated pretty well with the death rate. So we do not wish to imply that alcohol is in any way an essential ingredient of our diet: It is not. On the contrary, the effects of alcohol are potentially lethal: Cirrhosis of the liver, caused by excessive alcohol consumption, is the third most common cause of death among those aged 25–64 in New York City and other urban areas. We cannot do better than to conclude with a quotation from the English writer G. K. Chesterton, author of the Father Brown detective stories: "The dipsomaniac and the abstainer both make the same mistake: they both regard wine as a drug and not a drink."

There is much debate as to the optimal balance between fat and carbohydrate intake. Food fads recommend one thing, nutritionists another. A current fad suggests that one should not mix protein with carbohydrate or fat but should eat each separately; this seems nonsensical and there is no good evidence to support it. Currently carbohydrate is in, and fat is out. But it should be remembered that carbohydrate is turned into fat in the body anyway, and that some fat is essential because dietary triglyceride contains certain essential fatty acids that the body cannot synthesize from glucose, and because fat brings with it the fat-soluble vitamins A, D, E, and K. Then there is the argument that plant fat (e.g., margarine) is better than animal fat (e.g., butter) because it contains a higher proportion of unsaturated fatty acids (see Figure 10 in Chapter 2), and in any case butter contains cholesterol. But olive oil, another plant fat, is said to be even better than margarine: look at all those long-lived Mediterraneans. All this is no doubt true, but how relevant is it? The fact is that nutritional advice is often like ladies' fashions: For a period of time, long skirts are in; then fashion changes back to short skirts again, and so on. The analogy between ladies' fashions and our body is not so fanciful. In 1997 the Institute of Contemporary Arts in London mounted a fashion collection based on the molecular biology of the first 1000 hours of fetal development. Thirty-five different outfits were designed to represent successive stages of development, culminating in the appearance of the spinal column on day 42: This was represented by a silver-plated halter on a red dress depicting the way that the human genome is currently being analyzed. Our changing attitudes to nutrition are reflected in the way that one day dietary fiber in the form of spinach or potato skin is the hero and eggs the villain, while on another day fresh fish and seafood, previously shunned because of the possibility of mercury poisoning, are suddenly in. We are not saying that all of these recommendations are not based on experimental evidence of one sort or another, but as the sum total of knowledge increases, so certain previously held views become no longer tenable.

Take the case of radioactivity. My father used to travel once a year, for several decades after the end of World War II, to "take the waters" in a German spa (he was of a generation that still believed strongly in the therapeutic benefits of that kind of thing, and actually spas seem to be coming back—full cycle—into fashion). The point is that the spa advertised its waters as being beneficial because they were especially high in radioactive minerals, even though this was some years after atomic bombs had been dropped on Hiroshima and Nagasaki and the damaging effects of radioactive fallout had begun to be appreciated. Today the owner of the spa would probably be prosecuted if he admitted to his waters containing high amounts of radioactivity (most likely the spa continues to function; it's just the brochures that are different). The reason for telling this story is not to deny that radioactivity is a very serious health hazard (though my father lived to be 97), but to make an important point that applies particularly to nutrition: People are individuals, and some people may be more sensitive to the effects of undesirable foods than others. Equally, some people will benefit more from certain foods—high-vitamin-containing ones, for example—than others. Another way of putting it is that individuals vary very much from the mean. If one studies a sufficiently high number of people, one sees trends that are not evident in individuals. That is what statistics is about. There is absolutely no doubt that smoking is bad for our health and that it hastens death through heart disease and cancer. The fact that Winston Churchill, a lifelong smoker of cigars, lived into his 90s is irrelevant insofar as the overall population is concerned (in any case, the cigar in his mouth was often not lit). Statistically, then, what is the current advice regarding the type of food we should be eating? In simple terms it is this: high carbohydrate, low fat—especially low saturates—and high fiber. I shall return to the *amount* of food, in terms of calories, shortly.

Having preached, for the better part of 80 pages, the unity of molecular structure in all living species—let alone human beings—the author will now be accused of inconsistency. This would be unwarranted. Of course all human beings metabolize protein, fat, and carbohydrate in precisely the same way, and burn it up or store it in precisely the same way. What varies is the relative amount that is burned or stored. Just as no two human beings are alike in looks, so no two human beings are alike in the degree to which one metabolic pathway is followed compared with another one, or in the degree to which one person as opposed to another is susceptible to the common cold or to mild food poisoning. Unfortunately we do not yet know the molecular details of why one person will lose weight on a particular diet and another not, though we can assume that one way or another a subtle difference in proteins is involved. Two examples—unrelated to diet—illustrate this very point. It has been known for several decades that the molecules that are most varied between different individuals are a family of proteins known as the major histocompatibility complex (MHC) or human leukocyte antigens

(HLA). It is these proteins that play a role in graft rejection when tissues or organs are transplanted between people who are not identical twins. The relationship of these proteins to an individual's susceptibility to certain diseases, based on epidemiological studies, has long been suspected; a few years ago an example of a direct link was obtained. This concerned the observation that some people seemed to be resistant to developing malaria when bitten by *Plasmodium*-containing insects, whereas others from the same region succumbed to the disease; the molecular explanation of this observation in terms of MHC proteins is described in Chapter 5. A quite different reason why some people may develop a particular disease while others do not, is that the latter have in their cells an enzyme that inactivates the disease-causing molecule. The relationship between smoking and lung cancer provides a good and—in respect of the earlier remarks about Winston Churchill's cigars—a pertinent example. It has recently been found that smokers who have not developed lung cancer have in their tissues an enzyme (glutathione transferase) that detoxifies some of the carcinogenic molecules present in tobacco tar; those who do not have the enzyme—because they lack the appropriate gene—are more likely to develop lung cancer. So far as diet and other treatments are concerned, for the time being scientists and physicians have no choice but to study their effects on as large a sample of the population as possible, make their deductions, and then offer advice that will be applicable to the *average* person.

This does not mean that we should disregard all medical advice, since it might not apply to us. We would be foolish not to take penicillin if we have pneumonia or to refuse antimalarials if traveling to a malaria-infested zone, or to smoke two packs of cigarettes a day and wash them down with a bottle of Scotch. But to worry about the occasional pat of butter or slice of cream cake, if that is what makes one happy, is unfounded—provided, of course, one is not in a high-risk category such as being grossly overweight or having had three heart attacks already. Consider the following. Humans have been eating a pretty varying diet over the last 2000 years; the rich out of choice, the poor out of necessity. Yet the average life span of people over the age of 30 has not risen that much since Roman times: Our relatively unhealthy high-fat diet today is probably offset by better sanitation and health care. Under 30, the life span has increased phenomenally, because we are no longer dying of infectious diseases, especially in infancy; those who had reached 30 at the time of Julius Caesar had probably developed a pretty good immunity against the prevalent infectious diseases, even if they were not immune to having a knife stuck in their back. But nor are the peoples of the twentieth century immune to being slaughtered by the likes of Hitler, Stalin, Pol Pot, or Radovan Karadicz. If a person eats a sensible quantity of food, it does not matter too much what he eats: A calorie is a calorie whether it be protein, fat, or carbohydrate. But, as indicated above, we cannot simply dispense with one or other of these nutrients.

A certain amount of fat is essential because it contains necessary ingredients like vitamins A, D, E, and K and some unsaturated fatty acids that the body cannot synthesize. Some carbohydrate is essential because the body cannot turn fat into carbohydrate. This is because we—in common with all other animals—do not possess the enzymes for it; we do possess enzymes for turning carbohydrate into fat. And we all need protein because it is our major source of nitrogen and amino acids. We can synthesize most of the 20 amino acids from glucose, but we lack the enzymes to make the rest. Nucleic acids, as it happens, can be made entirely from carbohydrate and protein. Because of the extreme importance of proteins in the body as enzymes and structural molecules—fats and carbohydrate are in the main just fuels for energy—protein malnutrition is a severe defect. The infants picked up off the streets of Calcutta by Mother Theresa's Sisters of Charity are half the size of those from better homes, and will never catch up completely. Worse, they suffer irreparable brain damage, because the brain cells, once they are laid down in late pregnancy and early infancy, do not divide. It may in passing be noted that in this regard brain cells are to be contrasted with the cells of liver or the alimentary tract, which do divide. If, for example, a major part of the liver is removed surgically for lifesaving reasons, healthy cells in the remaining part will gradually divide to make up the

deficit. That is why some clinicians advocate the use of pig
liver transplants over human liver in certain cases of liver failure (the organs of pigs being roughly the same size as the organs of humans): The fact that the pig liver will start to be
rejected in time does not matter, because the residual human
cells will eventually grow to full size. If one of the kidneys is
removed surgically—sometimes for no better reason than to
donate it to a close relative in a critical condition—the remaining kidney will grow to larger than normal size in compensa-
tion. In short, the grossly undernourished infant may, if fed
properly, develop normal liver and kidney function, but his
mental capacity will remain retarded; his bones, too, will remain undersize. The importance of a balanced diet may be
seen if one compares the average size of Japanese over 50 with
those who are under this age. The old have the traditionally
short stature, but the young are surprisingly tall, because of
dramatic changes of diet after World War II. Do not suppose
that change of stature is related to a genetic change: Such
changes become manifest only over tens of thousands of years,
not decades. So who is to say that Texans are not taller because
their mothers fed them steaks from an early age? But there may
be another way for mothers to have their children growing up
to be tall: ensure that they are born in the spring. A recent
study over 10 years of half a million conscripts in Austria
showed that those born at the beginning of April are, on average, a quarter of an inch taller at the age of 18 than their counterparts born at the beginning of October. Overall, those born
between January and July are an eighth of an inch taller than
those born between July and December. While these differences may not be large—though remember they are only *averages*—they are highly significant. Astrologers the world over
will feel vindicated by these results. Have they not always told
us that our fate is dictated by the stars and the moon, by the
month in which we are born? We, however, must look for a
molecular explanation. The most likely is that the level of sunlight during the later weeks of pregnancy and the earliest
weeks after birth affects the subsequent growth of the child.
In Austria, as in many parts of the United States, the winter

months are cloudier than the spring ones. Light, we already know, affects the production of the hormone melatonin. Jet lag, for example, which is caused by a change in the periods of light and dark, reflects a disruption in the rhythm of melatonin formation, and some air travelers take extra melatonin to overcome this problem. The hypothesis is that melatonin somehow affects the growth rate at key moments in fetal and newborn life. An alternative explanation focuses on solar radiation, rather than on solar light itself. Solar radiation in the northern hemisphere is known to be maximal in July, and if radiation were somehow to improve egg quality at ovulation and conception, this could also explain the results, since children born in April are conceived in the previous July.

The reader is entitled—in a chapter on "The Healthy Body: Nutrition and Metabolism"—to *some* nutritional advice. I have already mentioned the benefits of carbohydrate and fiber over fat, of unsaturates over saturates. The relationship between body weight and caloric intake is disarmingly simple: If you ingest more calories than your body burns up (i.e., oxidizes glucose, fatty acids, and amino acids to CO_2 and H_2O), you will gain weight. This is because the extra calories will be deposited— largely as fat—within the body. If caloric intake equals caloric expenditure, the weight will stay the same. So we come to the vexed question posed by the overweight as to how they may best lose weight. By exercise, or by diet? The numbers of calories used up by different types of exercise are shown in Table 1. It is clear that you have to do an awful lot of exercise to burn up significant amounts. Much better to diet. Of course the ideal is to do both, since exercise tones up the muscles and keeps you fit during your dietary regime. What is considered as overweight? We are concerned here with the "clinically" obese; clinically, because obesity puts one at greater risk of developing hypertension (high blood pressure), heart disease, and diabetes (failure to metabolize carbohydrate properly with attendant consequences). We are not concerned here with people who wish to lose weight simply because they do not like their present figure. A good definition of obesity is related to the body mass index as follows. Measure your weight (in kilograms); then divide it by the square of your

Table 1. Caloric Expenditure and Content in Food

Activity	Energy expenditure
Resting	1650 calories/day (basal level)
Additional energy required for:	
Walking slowly for 1 hour	190 calories
Swimming for 1 hour	480 calories
Running for 1 hour, or walking upstairs for ½ hour	570 calories
Typing or ironing for 5 hours	720 calories
Carpentry or metalworking for 5 hours	1200 calories
Sawing wood for 3 hours	1385 calories
Mental activity for 5 hours	< 20 calories
An average working person might therefore expend a total of	2900 calories/day

Food	Caloric content
100 g (3.5 oz) of fat	950 calories
100 g of carbohydrate	400 calories
100 g of protein	400 calories
A daily diet of 50 g fat, 500 g (1 lb) carbohydrate, and 100 g protein would therefore provide	2900 calories/day

Adapted from *An Introduction to Human Biochemistry* by C. A. Pasternak, Oxford University Press, 1979.

height (in meters). This is known as the body mass index and gives a better measure of obesity than relating weight simply to height, because it correlates better with the actual amount of body fat. If your weight, for example, is 155 lb or 67.2 kg and your height is 5 feet 7 inches or 1.71 m, then your body mass index is 67.2 divided by 1.71 × 1.71, or 22.9. A body mass index of greater than 27.8 for men and 27.3 for women is defined as obese.

Obesity, like most diseases, is related to a combination of genetic and other causes. In the case of obesity, "other" means largely diet and exercise. The genetic causes are beginning to be unraveled: A protein called leptin that is secreted from adipose cells and acts on the appetite centers of the brain (the reader will recall Pavlov's experiment with salivating dogs) may be involved. Genetically engineered mice that are obese have much lower levels of leptin in their blood than their normal counterparts, and recently two related and severely obese children were found to have very low levels of leptin in their blood too. At the time of writing, evidence that decreased levels of leptin correlate with obesity in adults is lacking. Nevertheless the identification of a particular protein target opens up the possibility of designing drugs to boost leptin production, to substitute for leptin, to prevent leptin degradation, and so forth. It is knowledge of obesity at the molecular level that should give hope to obese individuals in the future.

So far as diet and exercise are concerned, then, the message is obvious: Eat less and exercise more. Exercising is essential, as otherwise the body tends to compensate for the decreased caloric intake by becoming lethargic, with the result that the adipose cells do not break down their fat (triglyceride) because there is no demand from the muscles for it. However, the relation between how many calories are burned and how many retained in the body is different in different people: Some burn up more even without much exercise, while others burn up less even when exercising. Do not be put off if a substantial initial weight loss is not maintained. The initial loss is probably unrelated to body fat. Body fat is lost rather slowly, but perseverance in reduced caloric intake, especially when coupled to exercise, will be rewarded. Remember, there are no obese survivors from labor camps.

As has just been pointed out, if you want to lose weight, eat less and exercise more. If you want to gain weight, eat more. Severely underweight individuals, though not common in the affluent countries of North America, Europe, and the Far East, are even more at risk from disease than obese people. In this case the most prevalent cause is infection. Malnutrition lowers the body's ability to fight disease, because the immune system is severely impaired. One has only to look at the starving masses of Somalia, Rwanda, and other parts of Africa. Whether the children one sees dying in the thousands, on our television screens from time to time, succumb to malnutrition or infectious disease is academic: They would not be in this condition if they had been fed properly. What is not academic is the criminality of the so-called politicians who deliberately drive communities from their farmlands and destroy the country's agriculture.

What of the vitamins and the trace minerals—iron, copper, zinc, and iodine—that play so important a role in the molecular reactions that occur in our cells? The role, incidentally, is analogous to the catalytic function of enzymes. In principle, therefore, they should not need replacing in an adult. Indeed, studies carried out in Oxford on students during the last war to try to determine the necessary dose of vitamin A for the British public failed because none of the students on a diet deficient in vitamin A developed any symptoms of deficiency! Coming from fairly affluent families, they had built up a sufficient reserve to make additional vitamin A unnecessary, at least over the period of the experiment. The situation would have been very different if children in Calcutta or Delhi had been studied: Vitamin A deficiency is common in India, where almost half of the population is living close to poverty and malnutrition; the same is true of the poor countries of Africa. In short, vitamins and trace minerals do leak out of the body in small amounts, and like enzymes that become degraded and need to be replaced by protein synthesis, so vitamins and trace minerals need to be replaced by including them in the diet. What doses of vitamin supplement and other goodies should we be taking? The answer, for an average person eating healthy food, is none: There is sufficient of everything in normal food. Breakfast cereals alone, as the manufacturers are keen to point out, contain most of the vitamins—at least the water-soluble B vitamins—that are necessary. And if your breakfast is limited to a cup of coffee or an orange juice, don't worry; you will ingest sufficient of these vitamins with your lunchtime sandwiches. Of course a pregnant woman, or one who experiences particularly heavy menstrual periods, should supplement her diet with iron and folic acid, required for making more red blood cells. In fact, up to 20% of women in North America and Western Europe suffer from anemia related to iron deficiency, and the figure reaches 60%—including children—in poorer countries. But most of the capsules, lozenges, ointments, juices, and other elixirs that are on offer are unnecessary and a waste of money. If you are convinced that they will make you feel better, preserve the moisture in your skin, increase your sexual potency, or whatever, by all means take them. They are unlikely to do harm except in megadoses, and insofar as a positive mind is beneficial to health, as discussed in Chapters 6 and 7, they are of benefit to those who believe in them.

Although a healthy person eating a mixed and varied diet should not need to supplement it with vitamins and minerals, this is not necessarily true for someone who is ill. Mention has been made of vitamin C for colds, and a similar claim has been made for zinc. Given that there is as yet no other remedy on offer (we are still waiting for a vaccine), there is no reason not to try these additives. And of course people who suffer from—albeit very rare—deficiency diseases that are the result of a genetic defect to absorb a necessary nutrient, should definitively supplement their intake. Pernicious anemia, resulting from an inability to absorb vitamin B_{12}, is an example. Acrodermatitis enteropathica, which is a rare skin ailment resulting from an inability to absorb zinc, is another. Interestingly, a quite different cause of the latter disease recently came to light. A patient with cancer of the bowel was on parenteral nutrition: all water and food—largely glucose, protein, and salts—administered through a drip directly into the bloodstream. Gradually the patient began to exhibit the symptoms of acrodermatitis enteropathica. It was the patient's husband who recognized these for what they were, discovered that there was no zinc in the solution being drip-fed, and persuaded the medical team to include this: The symptoms disappeared.

Here we have explored three of the major organs in the human body, the heart, kidneys, and liver, with passing reference to muscle, lungs, and the intestine. The aim has been to outline—at the molecular level—how the food that we eat is converted into energy, and the role that each of these organs plays in the process. The emphasis has been on the healthy body, and the stage is therefore set to consider in greater detail the causes of disease.

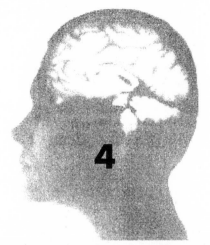

4

CAUSES OF DISEASE

GENES AND THE ENVIRONMENT

A ll disease has one of two causes: the genes or the environment (Table 2). In general, the more severe the consequences of a missing or faulty gene are, the rarer is the incidence. This is because those afflicted with a severely debilitating disease tend not to raise a family and therefore do not pass the gene on to the next generation. This is particularly true of the diseases that lead to death before maturity. Such "bad" genes are maintained in the population only because they are passed on by carriers.

Other diseases are predominantly environmental. They include nutritional disorders like malnutrition or iodine deficiency (in some regions of the Alps); pollutant disorders like silicosis (from asbestos inhalation), asthma (13% of cases in the urban population of Europe are probably the result of pollution), and some cases of leukemia (from radioactive fallout); stress-related illness; and the entire spectrum of infectious diseases. These range from infestation by protozoa (single-celled organisms such as the malarial parasites *Plasmodium vivax* and *Plasmodium falciparum*)

Table 2. Causes of Disease

Examples of diseases with predominantly genetic causes
  Hemoglobinopathies
  Hemophilia
  Tay–Sachs disease
  Cystic fibrosis

Diseases with predominantly environmental causes
  Nutritional
    Obesity
    Vitamin deficiency
  Pollution
  Stress
  Infection
    Measles
    Influenza
    Herpes
    HIV
    Tuberculosis
    Pneumonia
    Malaria
    Leishmaniasis

Examples of diseases with both genetic and environmental causes
  Heart disease
  Stroke
  Cancer
  Diabetes
  Asthma

---

and metazoa (many-celled organisms such as ringworm and tapeworm), through fungal or yeast infections *(Candida)*, and bacterial infections like blood poisoning (*Staphylococcus aureus, Clostridium*), food poisoning (*Salmonella, Escherichia coli, Vibrio cholerae*), diseases of lung (*Streptococcus pneumoniae, Mycobacterium tuberculosis*) or brain (*Meningococcus*), to viral infections of the respiratory system (influenza, whooping cough, common cold), nervous system (polio), immune system (human immunodeficiency virus— HIV), liver (hepatitis), genitals and other organs (herpes), and prion diseases like Creutzfeldt–Jakob disease. But in many common diseases like diabetes, cancer, arthritis, heart attack, or stroke, the contributions of genetic and environmental factors are more evenly balanced.

The relative effects of environment and genetic makeup on our bodies are graphically illustrated in relation to diet. As mentioned in the last chapter, an altered diet has increased the height of the Japanese population—whether in Japan or in the United States. But the other features, like skin coloration or shape of eyes, remain unaltered over hundreds of generations. Nor do Africans who have lived in Europe or the United States for many generations change their features any more than Europeans who have lived in Africa (the Boers, for example). Any dilution of features is related to intermarriage—a shuffling of genes at each generation—not to the environment. Eating a protein-rich diet, taking anabolic steroids, may make *you* tall and strong, but it will not affect your children. This is because the environmental effect is on various parts of the body like muscles and heart, not on the cells that are passed on to the next generation, namely, eggs in the ovaries and sperm in the testes. This is true even if the interaction is with the genes of heart or muscle. But if the environmental influence is one that causes DNA damage in general, like radioactive fallout, it will not discriminate between the DNA in heart or muscle and that in germ cells, that is, ovary or testis. The result in that case is that damage *is* passed on to the next generation. The higher incidence of Down's syndrome in children born to mothers over age 40 is an example that will be discussed shortly.

How, then, *do* characteristics like skin pigmentation gradually change over time, if—as scientists now say—it is likely that all species of *Homo sapiens* are descended from a single group of individuals? In short, how does Darwin's theory of evolution, namely, the concept of "survival of the fittest" (whether animal or man), work? The following discussion refers to *Homo sapiens*. The Neanderthal man that was for some time thought to be our direct ancestor probably is not. For there is evidence that both Neanderthalers and *Homo sapiens* coexisted for some of the time between 500,000 and 100,000 years ago. These dates for the emergence of man are relatively recent. A mere 50 years ago, when I was a boy, I recall reading in the science book of the day (by G. P. Wells) that "man is 30,000 years old." Imagine my surprise when, some years later, I visited the archaeological museum in Baghdad (having gone there to help Mustansiriyah University—a noble seat of learning for the best part of this millennium—to set up a medical school), only to find some beautiful man-made artifacts dated to more than 30,000 years ago. Whether Neanderthalers just died out because they could not cope with the climate or with the fierce animals around them, or whether they were gradually killed off by *Homo sapiens* because the latter found them an easier prey than some of the wild animals around at that time, or whether *Homo sapiens* outcompeted them for food and shelter, remains to be established. Certainly the success of *Homo sapiens* over his immediate nonhumanoid ancestors, the great apes, appears to reflect not his greater skill at hunting, but the exact opposite: because he was better at avoiding danger—running away from a fierce animal, not chasing it.

How did the different races of *Homo sapiens* evolve? Imagine a group of *Homo sapiens* of more or less similar coloring, stature, and so forth, living in East Africa around 150,000–250,000 years ago. (There are also suggestions that man evolved in the Far East, but the "out of Africa" theory remains the best bet.) Some of these remained in Africa, others gradually migrated to the northern hemisphere in what is now Europe and the western parts of Asia; others wandered farther, into the eastern parts of Asia; yet others found their way—who knows how—to Australia, New Zealand, and some of the islands of the Pacific (Figure 32). Those members of the group who remained in Africa, whose skin coloring was slightly darker than that of their fellows because of a higher concentration of the pigmented molecule melanin in their skin (remember no two individuals are exactly alike, because of slight differences in their DNA caused by random mutations), were at a marginal advantage because the strong rays of the sun did not affect them so much. Maybe fewer died of skin cancer. Gradually, over thousands of generations, those of darker coloring outbred their lighter-colored neighbors. I have chosen skin pigmentation as an example of a molecular characteristic of our bodies that does better in one environment as opposed to another, simply because it is more obvious to the observer. Equally I could have chosen one of a myriad other molecular characteristics: the ability to live at higher altitudes, or to survive in malaria-infested regions, for example. We shall meet this outgrowing of

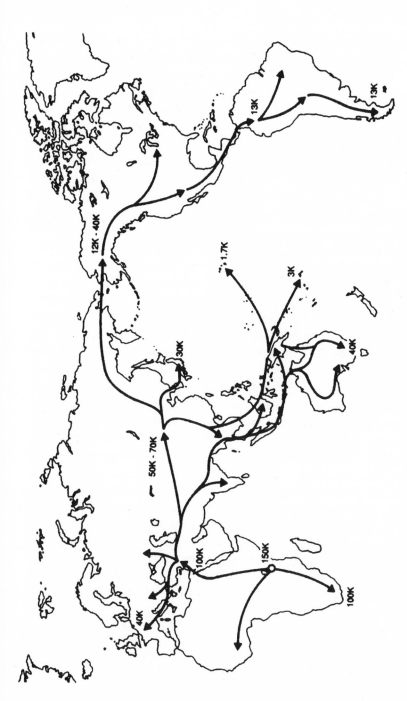

32. "Out of Africa." Speculative migration of human populations over the past 150,000 years (K = 1000 years). From M. Nei in *The Origin and Past of Modern Humans as Viewed from DNA* (edited by S. Brenner and K. Hanihara), World Scientific Publishing Co., 1995, with permission.

one population at the expense of others again: in the case of cancer cells exposed to chemotherapeutic drugs within our own body, where the time between generations is 24 hours (not 20–30 years), and in the case of bacteria exposed to an antibiotic, where the time between generations can be as short as 20 minutes. The principle of survival or selection of the fittest in a particular environment is the same.

In Europe and parts of Asia the opposite was occurring, and those who had migrated there became gradually lighter. It has to be said that the reasons why different racial groups developed different pigmentation is still very speculative. The skeletons of this period that have been found do not tell us much about the skin that covered them. All we can say is that the process of evolution is very slow, and for noticeable changes to appear takes tens of thousands of years, not just centuries. This, of course, does not take account of the mixing of genes through marriage. In that case altered characteristics like skin coloration appear already in the first generation. The point is that the reason why Africans, Asians, Europeans, the Aborigines of Australasia and the Pacific Islands, and the American Indians have retained their distinctive features over the past 50,000 years or so is just because they did *not* mix with each other and intermarry. Today, with more movement of people from one continent to another, more intermarriage and global air travel, the position is changing. Fifty thousand years from now, it is likely that all members of the species *Homo sapiens* will resemble each other as much as a Dutchman resembles a Belgian today.

The mechanism of evolution described here—selection of the fittest—has been challenged from time to time by a different theory: that environmental influences to which we are exposed *do* affect our offspring. A strong proponent of this view was Trofim Denisovich Lysenko who, during the 1930s and 1940s, used it to bolster communist dogma that the children of good communists will also be good communists because they will have inherited their parents' views. This theory obviously found favor with Stalin, even though later on he doubted—but only in private—the results of Lysenko's experiments. These concerned the growth of crops like wheat and rye. Lysenko appeared to provide evidence to show that the seeds of crops adapted to grow in a particular environment would inherit this ability. In short, that adaptation is hereditary. By the time he reached his heyday, just before Stalin's death in 1953, he was even claiming that wheat plants raised in the appropriate environment were able to produce seeds of rye. Attempts to repeat these experiments outside the Soviet Union failed, as did those within it (but these could not be published unless the authors were willing to languish in the labor camps of Siberia, or worse: Lysenko was a tyrant who did not tolerate opposing views). Inside the Soviet Union Lysenko's results inspired much of the thinking behind collective farming. We now know that collectivization was a monumental failure, and that millions of people starved because of it. Nevertheless Lysenko's influence on Soviet biology was so strong—especially on the appointment of professors and on what kind of results they could publish—that Soviet biology was held back for several decades and has only begun to recover significantly during the last 10 years.

Lysenko was not entirely without supporters in the West. Cyril Hinshelwood—an Oxford scientist who won the 1956 Nobel prize in chemistry for elucidating the details of chemical reactions like those between gaseous hydrogen and oxygen—was, like many misguided academics, an admirer of the Soviet system. Misguided in the sense that when such academics and other intellectuals visited Russia they were feted and shown just what the authorities decided the visitors should see: model schools, model hospitals, model collective farms, and, of course, a night out at the Bolshoi ballet. The visitors did not see villages—typical of the vast majority—in which peasants were living under conditions worse than during Tsarist times, nor did they see the labor camps of Siberia in which millions perished. Hinshelwood's scientific experiments, which purported to support Lysenko's views on adaptation, were on the mechanism by which bacteria become resistant to antibiotics. Bacteria can become adapted to growing in the presence of an antibiotic by the induction of an enzyme to destroy the antibiotic, as will be described in the next chapter. According to Hinshelwood, once a bacterium has adapted by the production of an enzyme, this ability to synthesize the enzyme is passed on to daughter cells. What all of the other experiments of the time—and since—showed was that bacteria do *not* pass on acquired characteristics in this way. Instead they show that a separate—mutant—line of cells, which outgrows the others in the presence of antibiotic, makes the enzyme irrespective of whether the antibiotic is present or not. (In fairness to Hinshelwood, it is possible that his observations were actually correct, but his interpretation wrong). We now know that bacteria acquire resistance to antibiotics directly from each other, that is, from already resistant strains. The way this happens is that one bacterium passes some of its genes—in the form of a small chromosome called a plasmid—to another bacterium. This process of shuffling antibiotic-resistant genes between one bacterial strain and another has become a major clinical problem. For it has resulted in the emergence of bacterial strains that have become resistant to every antibiotic currently available. If you have the misfortune to become infected with such a strain, you are in a very serious situation indeed. An infection of the lung, for example, leaves you in the same position as people were in half a century ago, before the discovery of antibiotics: That was when pneumonia was a killer not just for infants and the elderly, but for many an adult too.

We return to diseases caused by faulty genes (see Table 2 on p. 98). Disorders caused by a single gene defect are rather rare. They include diseases like Down's syndrome (severe mental retardation and abnormal appearance of face and limbs), thalassemias or sickle-cell disease (defective hemoglobin production), Huntington's disease (mental retardation), cystic fibrosis (accumulation of mucus in lungs and pancreas leading to malfunction and infection), hemophilia (failure to make the blood clotting factor VIII), and many others. Exactly how are such genetic defects, known as mutations, brought about? DNA is, like proteins, subject to wear and tear. The body is under constant bombardment from very low levels of background radiation such as radioactive radon gas emanating from the soil, from the ultraviolet rays of the sun, and from cosmic rays. Such radiations affect all molecules, through very slow, nonenzymatically catalyzed reactions, but nucleic acids are particularly prone to damage. Certain chemicals in food and in the environment, and the generation of free radicals (see Chapter 9) have a similar effect. Damage to DNA that is in the germ cells (ovaries in females, testes in males) is passed on to the next generation, whereas damage to a protein, or to DNA in any other type of cell, is limited to one generation only. Although the body has very efficient enzymes that detect and repair damaged DNA, very occasionally a fault in germ cell DNA is not rectified, and is then passed on to successive generations.

The fault may lie in the deletion of one or more of the nucleotides from a stretch of DNA or it may lie in the change of what was once, for example, an A into a G. Such faults (mutations) occur much more frequently if the mutagenic (causing mutations) background radiations increase for one reason or another. The leakage of radioactive fallout from the explosion at the Chernobyl nuclear power station in the Ukraine in 1986—the largest accidental release of radioactive material to date—is an example of a man-made increase. Natural increases in background rediation, due largely to radon gas, are insignificant. People who were living close to, or downwind of, the Chernobyl reactor developed an increased incidence of thyroid cancer (from radioactive iodine in the atmosphere: iodine is concentrated in the thyroid gland) and infant leukemia. More importantly, children born 6 years after the accident to parents who had been living within 200 miles of Chernobyl, were found to have a rate of mutation in a part of their DNA that is double the norm (some parts of the genome have higher mutation rates than other parts). However, it has to be said that such increases in mutation rate have not been found in offspring from the survivors of the atomic bombs dropped on Hiroshima and Nagasaki in 1945 (even though many survivors themselves subsequently died of thyroid cancer, leukemia, and other cancers caused by the radioactive molecules that had gotten inside their bodies).

The effect that a mutation causes depends on exactly where in the DNA of our chromosomes it occurs (Table 3). If it occurs outside a region coding for protein (i.e., a gene), it may have no effect and be, in essence, a "silent" mutation; on the other hand, it

Table 3. Effect of Mutations in DNA

Type of mutation	Effect	Example
Outside a gene	None	
Outside a gene at a control region	Reduced or increased amount of protein made	Thalassemias
Inside a gene	No protein made	Hemophilia, Tay–Sachs disease
Inside a gene	Faulty protein made	Sickle-cell disease, cystic fibrosis, many types of cancer
Exchange of piece of DNA between one chromosome and another	Various consequences	Certain types of cancer, especially leukemia
Extra chromosome made (3 copies, not 2)	Various consequences	Down's syndrome

may affect the control region for the synthesis of a protein, which may then be synthesized in reduced (or increased) amounts. This is the situation in the thalassemias, a group of blood disorders in which the hemoglobin of red cells is faulty. In α thalassemia, no A chains are made and the hemoglobin is made up of four B chains instead of being made up of two A chains and two B chains (see Figure 19 in Chapter 2); red cells containing this hemoglobin have a shorter life span, resulting in mild anemia. In β thalassemia, hemoglobin with two gamma chains and two B chains are formed; this does not bind oxygen so well, which is therefore not delivered to the tissues properly. The diseases are prevalent among Mediterranean populations, which explains their name: *thálassa* is Greek for "sea," and to the Greeks there was only one sea, namely, the Mediterranean. In diseases such as hemophilia, phenylketonuria, Tay–Sachs disease, or lactose intolerance, the protein is not made at all. In the case of the last three examples, the protein is an important enzyme of metabolism. The protein is not made either because of a mutation in the control region outside its gene, or because of a mutation at the start of its gene. In phenylketonuria the missing enzyme is one that is involved in the breakdown, to carbon dioxide and water, of phenylalanine, which is one of the 20 amino acids present in proteins. As a result, phenylketone molecules accumulate and spill over into the urine (-*uria* means "pertaining to urine"; -*emia* means "pertaining to blood," as in anemia, leukemia, hypercholesterolemia, and so on). Accumulation of phenylalanine and phenylketone is toxic, especially to brain. In Tay–Sachs disease the missing enzyme is one involved in the breakdown of certain lipids, which therefore accumulate; again toxicity is greatest in brain. In lactose intolerance the missing enzyme—in many cases just not enough enzyme—is one that breaks down lactose (to glucose and galactose; see Chapter 2); the enzyme is situated in the wall of the intestine where it enables lactose from food to be absorbed. The treatment for lactose intolerance is simple: Avoid milk. The treatment for phenylketonuria is more difficult: Instead of eating protein, eat a purified mixture of the 20 amino acids, with the amount of phenylalanine kept minimal. There is currently no treatment for Tay–Sachs disease.

In diseases such as sickle-cell disease (Figure 33) or cystic fibrosis, protein *is* made, but just one of its amino acids is substituted for by a different one because of a mutational change in the triplet that codes for the amino acid at that position. In sickle disease, for example, the amino acid glutamate at position 6 of the B chain of hemoglobin is replaced by the amino acid valine at the same position, as a result of a mutation in the triplet GAG, coding for glutamate, to the triplet GTG, coding for valine—in other

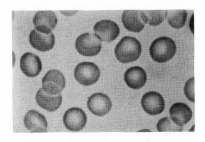 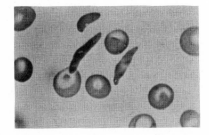

33. Sickle cells. (Left) Normal red blood cells (containing hemoglobin A). (Right) Mixture of normal and sickle cells (containing hemoglobin S). Courtesy of Dr. P. T. Flute. From *An Introduction to Human Biochemistry* by C. A. Pasternak, Oxford University Press, 1979.

words, a mutation, from A to T, in just one out of some 500 nucleotides in the gene for the B chain of hemoglobin. The outcome of such mutations is that the proteins function less effectively, if at all. We may compare the function of proteins to that of a subway train. If just one door, out of more than 50 on an average train, fails to shut, the train will not start. But if the seats of an entire car are ripped out (more difficult to achieve with the wooden seats in New York than with the upholstered ones in Washington, D.C. or London, England), it has no effect whatsoever on the ability of the train to move. So it is with proteins. Entire regions can be missing or faulty without any effect on the ability of the protein to carry out its function. But if a single amino acid in a crucial part— such as the active site of an enzyme, or the site near the heme of hemoglobin—is altered, the entire protein fails to function.

In some diseases the change in DNA is not so subtle. In certain types of cancer, for example, an entire portion of one chromosome is transferred to another chromosome; although all of the genes are still intact, the genes in the translocated part now come under the control of the new region to which they have been joined, and more or less of the respective proteins are made. In Down's syndrome, to be described shortly, the genetic change is even more dramatic. Again, all genes are present, but chromosome number 21 (see Figure 14 in Chapter 2) is present as three copies instead of two. How such an imbalance of chromosome number leads to the symptoms of Down's syndrome is still a mystery.

The effects of different mutations in DNA have been particularly closely studied in glucose-6-phosphate dehydrogenase (G-6-PD) deficiency. In this disorder an enzyme involved in glucose oxidation is affected (Figure 34). The oxidation (removal of hydrogen atoms) of glucose-6-phosphate—catalyzed by the enzyme G-6-PD—is linked to the reduction (addition of hydrogen atoms) of the small peptide glutathione. Glutathione is made up of three amino acids, one of which is the sulfur-containing amino acid cysteine. Cysteine, and as a result glutathione, exists in either the reduced form (a hydrogen atom, H, on the sulfur atom, S) or the oxidized form (no hydrogen atom, H, on the sulfur atom, S). Reduced glutathione is important in that it maintains the iron of

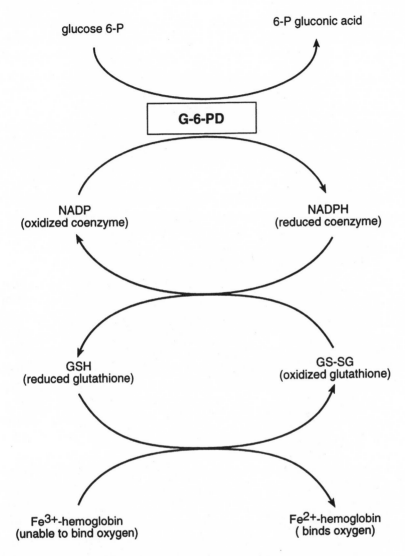

34. Biochemistry of G-6-PD deficiency.

heme in hemoglobin in the reduced (ferrous) state (Figure 35). Iron is an atom that has two valences: It is either in the reduced state, as in Fe^{2+} (ferrous), or in the oxidized state, as in Fe^{3+} (ferric). When the iron of hemoglobin is in the oxidized ferric state, oxygen can no

35. Oxygen binding by hemoglobin. The heme part of hemoglobin, which is linked to the protein part (globin), is shown without oxygen (upper panel) and with oxygen (lower panel). The iron atom (Fe) is seen in the center of the ring structure known as *porphyrin*. From *An Introduction to Human Biochemistry* by C. A. Pasternak, Oxford University Press, 1979.

longer bind to it; this is what happens to blood when it is left standing about for a long time: The red color of hemoglobin gradually darkens and becomes almost black as the iron is oxidized to the Fe^{3+} state; the same happens to a cut or a graze on the skin.

The reader may consider it paradoxical that the oxygen (O_2) bound to hemoglobin (in its Fe^{2+} state) does not itself oxidize the iron to Fe^{3+}. But if it did, hemoglobin would be useless as an oxygen carrier, because there would be no oxygen left for the tissues if it was all used up (i.e., reduced, eventually to H_2O) by its reaction with hemoglobin. Evolution has gradually selected Fe^{2+}, attached to heme which is itself attached to globin as shown in Figure 35, as an ideal atom for binding O_2 without being oxidized by it. But this does require the presence of reduced glutathione to maintain the Fe^{2+} state. An alternative strategy for carrying oxygen in the blood evolved in some animals, like insects and mollusks: These bind oxygen to a copper-containing molecule (hemocyanin) instead; hence their blood is blue, not red. The origin of the term "blue blood" to describe persons of aristocratic lineage is not, however, meant to suggest their resemblance to snails or oysters. The term probably originated in Spain 500 years ago in order to distinguish Castilian nobles from lesser mortals, some of whom were of Semitic or Moorish origin: The veins of the fair-skinned Castilians seemed to look bluer than those of darker folk.

G-6-PD deficiency has been studied in considerable detail, and more than 300 different molecular variants—many with just a single amino acid substitution out of the 532 amino acids that constitute the protein—have been identified in different groups of people living predominantly in the subtropical and tropical areas of the Mediterranean, Africa, and Asia. In some cases the enzyme functions with less than 0.1% efficiency of normal; in some it functions with 100% efficiency, while in other cases it functions with intermediate values of efficiency. In some of the cases where the enzyme is 100% effective, an amino acid substitution makes the protein more susceptible to degradation—the wear and tear of proteins. In cells other than red cells, in which the protein is being continuously resynthesized, the defect is not so serious. But in red cells, where there is no machinery for protein synthesis, it means that the efficacy and life span of the cells is reduced, hence the anemia.

We now know that G-6-PD deficiency is the underlying cause of diseases previously termed favism—a disorder resulting from eating too many fava beans—and primaquine intolerance—a disorder brought on by the antimalarial drug primaquine. In each case a defective G-6-PD enzyme fails to metabolize a potentially toxic molecule properly: a constituent of the fava bean on the one hand and the molecule primaquine on the other hand. Why is G-6-PD deficiency so prevalent in some areas and not in others? One reason is that the presence of the enzyme in red cells makes it more difficult for the parasites that cause malaria—*Plasmodium vivax* and *P. falciparum*—to grow inside red cells. It is just in areas where the incidence of G-6-PD deficiency is high, that malaria is rife. A similar reason is likely to account for the incidence of sickle-cell disease (an abnormal hemoglobin, as explained above) in such areas. In short, a predisposition to one disease—like the malfunctioning of red cells—in certain populations is offset by their resistance to other diseases—like malaria. As a result, what is potentially a debilitating gene is retained at a relatively high level in the population. Many of the genes in our body that seem to be of little advantage today probably reflect the different environmental conditions to which our ancestors were subject 10,000 to 100,000 years ago. As already mentioned, inheritance of genetic mutations is a very slow process indeed.

By examining proteins like G-6-PD in the laboratory, it has become clear that mutations that do not alter the efficacy of a particular protein are very widespread. What, then, is "mutant" and what is "normal"? Where there is no difference in efficacy, the term "polymorphism" (Greek for "many forms") is used instead. In this case, "mutant" and "normal" have no meaning because they are equally functional forms of the same protein. After all, we do not speak of blue eyes as being a mutant form of brown eyes (or vice versa), nor do we refer to fair or red hair as being a mutant of dark hair.

Not all genetic diseases are inherited from our parents. Down's syndrome, for example, results from damage to the DNA while it is in the ovaries of the mother. If an egg containing damaged DNA becomes fertilized, it will develop into a baby containing damaged DNA. Why should the DNA of eggs in the ovaries become damaged? The reason is that the eggs within the ovary are all laid down around birth and are then released in turn at each menstrual cycle. They are therefore subjected to environmental damage (for example, chemical reactions like free radical formation, to be described in Chapter 9) for the entire life of the mother. Because such damage is cumulative, the older the mother is before she conceives, the greater the chance that the DNA of her eggs has become damaged. That is why women who conceive over the age of 40 are encouraged to have their fetus screened at the earliest opportunity so that they may—if they so wish—have an abortion should the fetus have Down's syndrome: The life of such a child, or that of its parents, is not an easy one. On the other hand, it has recently been found that women who live to the age of 100 or more are four times more likely to have had children during their 40s, than women who die at age 73; so having children late in life may be good for the mother, though not for her offspring. How about the prospective fathers of a Down's syndrome child? Are they not at least as likely as the mothers to have been the cause, especially as many men continue to be fertile well into their 70s? The answer is no, for the simple reason that sperm are not laid down in the testes at birth like eggs within the ovaries. Sperm are made anew after every ejaculation and do not therefore accumulate mutations in the way that eggs do.

Another example of a disease that has a genetic basis that is not necessarily inherited is cancer. Cancer, or rather the group of diseases that result from uncontrolled division of one cell type followed by spread to other organs and more generally referred to as malignancy, arises when a cell loses the mechanism that normally tells it to stop dividing; the result is unabated proliferation of the affected cell. What is that mechanism? There are, in fact, several, for there exist in all dividing cells various proteins that control cell division either positively (they promote it) or negatively (they inhibit it). In malignant cells the positive controls are augmented and the negative controls reversed. An example will illustrate one way by which this is achieved. One of the negative controls is p53, a protein that is being particularly extensively studied (over 3000 scientific publications on this protein alone between 1991 and 1996). One reason for this is that in about half of all types of cancer—including some of the commonest like carcinoma of breast, lung, and colon—the p53 molecule is found to have been altered by a mutation or deletion in the p53 gene. The effect in each case is to promote cell growth, and normal p53 has been called a tumor (cancer) suppressor molecule.

Several environmental causes for the mutation of genes like that for p53 have been proposed. Tar from cigarette smoking is one (the nicotine contained in cigarettes is not itself carcinogenic, but rather it is addictive, which is why the tobacco industry prefers to leave it in cigarettes). A third of all cancers result from smoking, as do 99% of cases of lung cancer. Half of all those who smoke will die as a result of smoking. A pack of cigarettes a day takes 8 years off your life; each cigarette shortens your life by 10 minutes. These figures include death from a heart attack as well as from cancer. The knowledge that it is the tar, not the nicotine, in cigarettes that is the killer has not reduced deaths from low-tar cigarettes. On the contrary, because people who smoke low-tar cigarettes inhale more, they too are coming down with the disease. Among 2 million people recently analyzed in Connecticut, there was a 17-fold increase in adenocarcinoma (one of the forms of lung cancer) in women between 1959 and 1991; the increase in men over the same period was 10-fold.

Infection with particular viruses is another cause of cancer. Although most viral infections do not affect the DNA of the cell to which they have gained access and in which they then multiply, in other types of virus, the viral DNA or a DNA copy of the viral RNA (viruses contain either DNA or RNA, never both) becomes integrated into the host DNA. That is, a stretch of the host DNA contains viral, not human, genes. One of these viral genes codes for a protein like p53, but because it is derived from a virus, the protein is not identical with human p53. One of the differences is that the viral p53 does not limit cell division, but promotes it. Thus do the molecules of viruses become lethal agents.

The story of a link between viruses and cancer actually began almost a century ago. In 1910 the American biologist Peyton Rous (Figure 36) was examining the causes of sarcoma (a cancer of connective tissue cells) in chickens. He found that he could transmit the disease from one chicken to another, which suggested to him that an infectious agent was at play. Rous went on to show that the infectious agent was a virus, which became

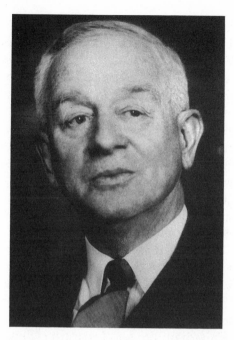

36. Peyton Rous. Nobel laureate, 1966. Half a century earlier, he had shown that a sarcoma (cancer) in chickens is caused by a virus. Copyright: The Nobel Foundation, Stockholm.

known as Rous sarcoma virus in his honor. Peyton Rous was one of the first scientists to study a virus in detail, and one of the first to propose a rational cause for cancer. But Rous was a man before his time: Half a century was to pass before scientists once again took up the idea that viruses could cause cancer.

Then, during the 1970s, the idea snowballed: It even reached the presidency of the United States. President Richard Nixon took up the fight against cancer with a vengeance. His predecessor John F. Kennedy had placed men on the moon; he, Richard Milhous Nixon, would find a cure for cancer. And a cure was a realistic goal, since we now knew that cancer could be caused by viruses. Millions of dollars were thrown into the fight; at one point Congress *increased* the budget requested by the National Cancer Institute—a quite unprecedented occurrence. And what happened? Several very exciting advances in unraveling the molecular details of viral growth and replication were made. Several scientists won Nobel prizes (Figure 37). But cancer? The number of people dying of cancer in the United States two decades after Nixon's crusade is virtually unchanged: Of the four most common causes of death, lung cancer deaths have actually increased, especially in elderly women as more young women started to smoke after World War II, and so have deaths from cancer of the prostate, while deaths from breast cancer are pretty much the same and only deaths from cancer of the bowel have decreased slightly (Table 4). The reason why death from cancer in the elderly appears to be increasing probably reflects the fact that management of heart disease has improved, so people are living longer and are therefore more likely to contract some form of cancer.

Of course it is true that it takes several years before a discovery in the laboratory can be introduced into the clinic, though there are notable exceptions. Diabetes was an incurable disease until 1921. It was known that sufferers could not absorb glucose properly from the bloodstream into tissues like muscle. In that year a Canadian, Frederick Banting (Figure 38), and his colleague Charles Best isolated a protein from pig pancreas that rectified the problem in experimental animals. Immediately

Table 4. Changes in Death Rates from Cancer, United States, 1973–1990

Cancer type	% increase (+) or decrease (–) in death rates (to nearest 10%)	
	Patients under 65	Patients under 65
Lung (females)	+70	+200
Lung (males)	0	+30
Breast (females)	–10	+10
Liver	+20	+20
Prostate	+10	+20
Bowel	–20	–10
Brain	–10	+70
Skin melanoma	+20	+70
Leukemia	–20	+10
Cervical cancer	–40	–40
Testicular cancer	–70	–70

Adapted from T. Beardsley, Scientific American, 270, 118, 1994.

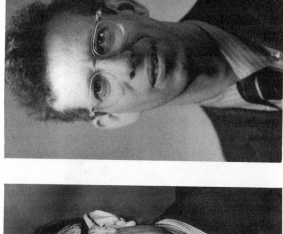
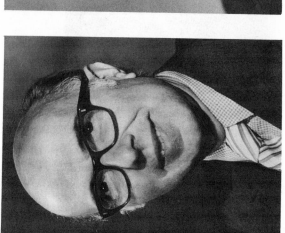
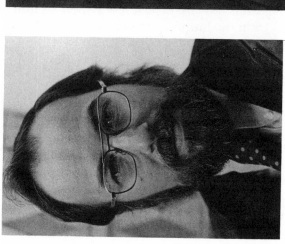

37. David Baltimore, Renato Dulbecco, and Howard Temin. Nobel laureates, 1975. From left to right: Baltimore, Dulbecco, and Temin. Between them they showed how tumor (cancer) viruses transform cells from normal to cancer by interacting with the DNA of normal cells. Copyright: The Nobel Foundation, Stockholm.

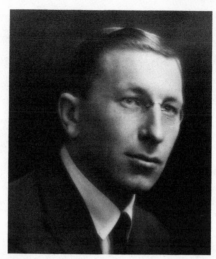

38. Frederick Banting. Frederick Banting (Nobel laureate, 1923) and Charles Best isolated insulin from pancreas. Copyright: The Nobel Foundation, Stockholm.

thereafter the pig protein, called insulin, was injected into human diabetics. A cure had been found. Well not exactly a cure, rather a treatment, since diabetics still required daily injections of insulin. But it was a landmark. It was the first identification of a hormone in molecular terms (that is, a protein) and it was the first time that a molecule derived from an animal was injected into human beings; it is only in the last few years that human insulin—prepared from the human gene introduced into bacteria, not from human pancreas—has become available. Although diabetes is a common disease that affects 1 in 10 of the population, only 10–20% of these require insulin (type 1 diabetes): Most can be treated by diet alone (type 2 diabetes). Another rapid advance happened 30 years later. Howard Florey, a pathologist, and Ernst Chain, a chemist (Figure 39), headed an Oxford team of scientists trying to isolate the active ingredient secreted by the mold *Penicillium notatum*. The reason for their efforts was that over a decade earlier, Alexander Fleming in London had shown that the ingredient, subsequently called penicillin, stops the growth of certain disease-causing bacteria like staphylococci. In 1940 came success. Pure penicillin was successfully isolated (and

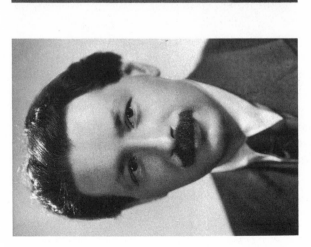
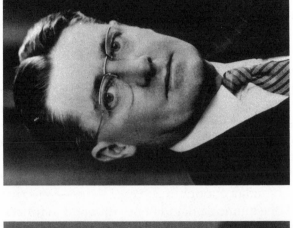

39. Ernst Chain, Alexander Fleming, and Howard Florey. From left to right: Chain, Fleming, and Florey. Fleming showed that the fungus (mold) *Penicillium notatum* secretes a substance that stops bacteria from growing. Chain and Florey isolated the substance (penicillin) and showed it to be effective against several infectious microbes. Copyright: The Nobel Foundation, Stockholm.

its molecular structure determined) from the culture fluid of *Penicillium notatum*. Within weeks Florey was injecting it into patients with blood poisoning. Another landmark: in this case the first isolation of an antibiotic and its use against bacterial infections. But landmarks are rare.

The main reason for the lack of progress in regard to cancer was that in only a very few cases could live viruses be isolated from cancer cells. The fact that viral genes can integrate themselves into host DNA, and then subvert the control mechanisms of the host cell into unrestricted growth were then not known; only today do we realize that proteins (e.g., p53) that are made by viral genes, are similar enough to host proteins—yet crucially different in just one amino acid and hence different in function—to cause cancer. In any case, even if cancers *are* caused by viruses, there was very little anybody could do about it, since very few drugs that are effective against viruses were known—or, for that matter, are known today. Cancer of the liver caused by hepatitis B virus may be an exception. People who have been infected with the hepatitis B virus are prone to develop liver cancer. Hepatitis B is prevalent in parts of Africa and Asia—particularly in southern China and southeast Asia—where up to 90% of the population is infected. The virus causes 1½ million deaths a year from liver failure. Because the virus is passed from an infected mother to her offspring, hepatitis B is now being diagnosed in considerable frequency in children born in the United States of immigrant Chinese parents. A vaccine developed against hepatitis B has proved effective at preventing hepatitis in children (it is pretty ineffective in adults). Over a 10-year period, starting in 1984, the incidence of liver cancer in 6- to 9-year-olds in Taiwan who were vaccinated as babies has fallen to a quarter. The aim now is to vaccinate all babies in high risk areas. At last perhaps, with all of the knowledge gained over the past 20 years, we may be on the threshold of developing effective therapies against cancer—the last of the killer diseases that is responsible for 20% of all deaths, yet that we have been unable to tame during the course of this century. (This, of course, is more or less what was said in the early 1970s.)

A discussion on the causes of cancer would be incomplete without mentioning two factors, the first of which is not related to a genetic change during the lifetime of an individual who develops a cancer. This is a genetic susceptibility that is inherited, and the second is the effect of diet. Many cancers run in families, and studies with populations of inbred mice show that some populations are many times more likely to develop cancers than others. Recently, two genes that are associated with susceptibility to breast cancer in women (who are 100 times more likely to develop the disease than men) have been described. The first is called BRCA 1, the other BRCA 2. Both genes have been detected in much greater proportion in breast cancer patients than in the rest of the population. The race to discover exactly what type of protein is made by the BRCA genes, and how such proteins transform breast cells into cancer cells, is on.

The second factor, diet, *may* cause cancer by acting on genes in certain cases. The following is just one example. An effect of diet was recognized several years ago when a relationship between spoiled food and liver cancer was established. The rogue molecules are protein toxins produced by molds (fungi) that bind to DNA and cause mutations; the molecule aflatoxin that is secreted by *Aspergillus* is one of such toxins. Other cases are less clear-cut and depend very much on epidemiological studies. Overeating—too many calories—is a risk factor not only for heart disease, but for cancer also. Breast cancer in women is a particularly common outcome. High fat diets likewise predispose to both heart disease and cancer. Again breast cancer in women is common, as is cancer of the colon and rectum in both sexes. Many other foods, and especially some food additives are suspected of being involved in the progression toward cancer. Additives that contain molecules capable of generating free radicals (to be discussed in Chapter 9) are particularly suspect. Frying foods in fat adds to the risk of fat alone, as frying promotes the formation of potentially carcinogenic (leading to cancer) molecules, since some of the products are known to bind to DNA. The reader will detect a noncommittal air about the dangers of food. This is merely because we lack hard evidence and it would be wrong to spread scare stories at this stage. What scientists are clear about is that a third of all cancers are related to diet, with another third related to tobacco. And remember that both diet and tobacco are also major risk factors for heart disease, and that cancer and heart disease account for well over half of all deaths.

There may also be good news on the food front. Vegetables like broccoli and Brussels sprouts contain "secondary compounds" that may be beneficial against cancer. These compounds, glucosinolates, act as antioxidants by mopping up free radicals that are potentially carcinogenic. So convinced are scientists of the benefits of glucosinolates that they are even introducing into other vegetables the enzyme that makes them, like cabbages, through genetic engineering techniques. A recent report suggests that drinking green tea may also have a beneficial effect in halting the spread of various kinds of cancer. The ability of malignant cells to invade a tissue remote from the site of the original tumor depends on the action of enzymes secreted by the malignant cells. These enzymes enable the cells to burrow their way out of the tissue of origin into the bloodstream, and out of the bloodstream back into other tissues. Green tea contains epigallocathechin-3 gallate (EGCG), a molecule that is a very complex derivative of carbolic acid. EGCG is now said to inhibit one of the enzymes secreted by malignant cells. The potentially therapeutic action of green tea deriving from its content of EGCG is but one instance of many such claims that appear in the scientific literature every week; and a year has 52 weeks. The databases of potential anticancer drugs are crammed with hundreds of thousands of compounds, very few of which have found their way into clinical practice once exhaustive trials have been conducted. I cite the case of EGCG merely because it illustrates the link between alternative or complementary medicine (drinking green tea is part of traditional Chinese medicine) and orthodox medicine, to which we shall return in a later chapter. Suffice it to say at this point that inhibitors of enzymes secreted by malignant cells have long been sought by pharmaceutical and biotechnology companies. A recent such compound patented by the U.K. company British Biotech Ltd., called marimastat, has hit the market. Let us hope that its results in the clinic are effective.

A fairly lengthy discussion of cancer seems warranted because it provides a good example of the interplay between genes and the environment in molecular terms. It also remains one of the most common, unpleasant and painful, and often drawn-out causes of death. Another example is heart disease. It is *the* most common cause of death and also involves both genetic and environmental risk factors. Although family studies have long pointed to a genetic predisposition toward heart disease, no culprit genes have yet been identified, except indirectly in relation to an abnormally high content of triglyceride or cholesterol in the bloodstream (hypertriglyceridemia and hypercholesterolemia are inherited disorders). On the other hand, epidemiological studies have clearly indicated a link with certain lifestyles. These include smoking (in this instance probably the nicotine as well as the tar), a sedentary lifestyle (insufficient exercise), obesity (excessive caloric intake), and a high consumption of fat (it must be remembered that although we produce triglyceride and cholesterol in our bodies anyway, eating excess is detrimental). Obesity itself has a genetic element in addition to the environmental one: A possible molecular explanation in terms of the protein leptin that controls appetite was given in the previous chapter.

A disease that until recently was thought not to depend on genetic factors at all is acquired immune deficiency syndrome (AIDS), caused by infection with HIV. More than 30 million people worldwide are currently infected with HIV, and over 60% of these are in Africa; the death rate there is currently some 8 million per year. Most of those infected with HIV go on to develop AIDS (a characteristic inability to fight off most types of infectious microbes) within a number of years and most eventually die of an infection they might otherwise have been able to shake off, or from certain cancers, especially lymphomas (proliferation of lymphocytes, one of the white cells in the bloodstream, in lymph nodes and in organs like thymus, tonsils, and spleen). Yet a few individuals seem never to develop AIDS, even though they clearly have HIV in their bloodstream. Why is this? The answer lies in the way the virus invades its target cell, namely, T4 cells (a class of lymphocytes). The virus has been known for some time to invade T4 lymphocytes because a protein on the viral surface happens to bind well to a protein on the surface of T4 lymphocytes. Having made such contact, the virus enters the cell by fusing its membrane with that of the lymphocyte. Once inside, it multiplies, is released from the lymphocyte, and goes on to invade other cells. What has recently been found is that a second protein on the surface of the T4 lymphocyte is required to participate in the binding between virus and lymphocyte in order for invasion by the virus to be successful. Analysis of the proteins on the surface of lymphocytes of the small number of individuals who are resistant to HIV infection shows that in their case the second protein is missing (or is present in altered form). As more molecular studies are carried out on people who appear to be resistant to some microbial infections, more examples of such genetic factors (since the type of proteins on the surface of cells are known to be inherited) are likely to emerge. A quite different mechanism of genetic resistance—in this case to malaria—will be described in the following chapter.

Earlier it was mentioned that males are more likely to develop the symptoms of certain genetic diseases than females. Why is this? Before proceeding to an answer, the nature of chromosomes must be briefly discussed. Practically every cell in the body contains 23 pairs of chromosomes, i.e., 46 in all (see Figure 14 in Chapter 2). Shortly before cell division, when a cell splits into two replica daughter cells, the DNA of each chromosome is doubled so that there are now 92 chromosomes; during cell division (called mitosis) the number of 46 chromosomes per cell is restored. The exceptions are red blood cells, which contain no chromosomes, and the cells of testis and ovary, which each contain just one set of 23; when sperm enters an egg cell in the act of fertilization, the number of 46 is restored. Every cell from then on will again have 46, one set of 23 paternal chromosomes and one set of 23 maternal ones. Each of the 23 chromosome pairs is different in length, and hence in genetic content; but within any one pair, the chromosomes are virtually identical in appearance; in genetic content, of course, they differ because one chromosome contains the genes inherited from the father, whereas its partner contains the genes inherited from the mother. This is true of 22 of the chromosomes, and of the 23rd pair in females; in males, the 23rd pair consists of one chromosome that resembles the female chromosome, called an X chromosome, and one chromosome that is much shorter, called a Y chromosome (Figure 14).

Whether an offspring is going to be male or female is a consequence of a process that begins in the testes. When the precursor cells of sperm—each containing 46 chromosomes with one X and one Y—divide, they do so without doubling the chromosomes first. Hence, half the sperm cells will contain an X, and half a Y chromosome. During ejaculation, some 300 million sperm are released and swim by means of a whiplike flagellum up the vagina toward the uterus (a lot of energy from glucose oxidation, transmitted via ATP, is used up in the process). Only a few (approximately 100) viable sperm make it to the site of an egg in the uterine tube; the rest die on the way. Those that make it swim around the egg like flies around a jar of honey. Eventually one sperm will penetrate the mucus layer that surrounds the egg (by means of enzymes released from the sperm head) and enter; immediately thereafter a barrier is created that prevents further sperm from entering the egg. If the successful sperm contains an X as its 23rd chromosome, it will produce a girl; if it contains a Y, it will produce a boy. Since exactly half of the many sperm on their way to the egg contain an X chromosome and half a Y chromosome, there is an equal chance of producing a boy or a girl. But some people do not like to let nature throw the dice. Obliging scientists are even now developing techniques for separating Y-containing sperm away from X-containing ones, so that, with appropriate *in vitro* fertilization techniques, the sex of an offspring can be virtually predetermined. Depending on one's moral view regarding abortion, an alternative—but less acceptable one in Western society—is to have the sex of the developing fetus analyzed, which can now be done at a very early stage of pregnancy, and proceed with an abortion if the offspring is not of the desired sex.

During protein synthesis, the DNA from each of the two chromosomes on which a particular gene is located, is read off and processed into protein. Half of the protein is therefore made from the paternal chromosome, half from the maternal one. Since most of the proteins in the body—hemoglobin, insulin, the enzymes of food degradation and oxidation, of ATP synthesis and utilization, and so forth—are the same in all human beings, all molecules of the synthesized protein are alike. But if a particular gene has a mutation in it, in either the paternal or maternal chromosome, a mixture of protein molecules is produced. (This assumes that the mutant gene produces a mutant protein; if it produces no protein at all, the total number of protein molecules produced is simply halved.) Such, for example, is the situation in sickle-cell disease (Figure 33): half of the hemoglobin molecules in the red blood cells are normal, half have one amino acid out of the 140 present changed and do not function properly. The disease is not too serious because 50% of normally functioning hemoglobin molecules is sufficient for carrying oxygen through the bloodstream under normal conditions. Such a mutation is known as recessive. (If both of the genes that are inherited are mutant, of course, the situation is much worse as there is now no normally functioning hemoglobin at all.) In contrast, some mutations are dominant. It requires a mutation in only one of the chromosomes to produce the severely debilitating mental disorder known as Huntington's disease: The protein produced by the mutant gene causes malfunctioning of brain cells even though its normal partner is present.

In the case of genes on the X and Y chromosomes, the situation is different. First, the Y chromosome contains no genes that are necessary for body processes; if essential genes were on the Y chromosome, females could not function properly, which is not the case. What the Y chromosome contains are some genes concerned with maleness, such as the genes for producing testes, which synthesize the male hormone testosterone; testosterone is also synthesized outside the testes, as females can have up to 10% as much testosterone in their bloodstream as males: The distinction between maleness and femaleness is obviously less clear-cut than many suppose (not so much Butch Cassidy as Butch Cassandra). How about the X chromosome, of which there are two in females and one in males? The X chromosome contains many genes that are required for normal body function. Females do not produce twice as much of the relevant proteins as males, because one of the X chromosomes is permanently inactivated in every cell so that none of its genes are transcribed into protein. Because the expression of genes on the X chromosome is the same in males as in females, it is thought that femaleness is the basic characteristic and that maleness is superimposed on it in males by the expression of genes—like those coding for the enzymes of testosterone synthesis—situated on the Y chromosome. In other words, males have all of the genes necessary for synthesizing female hormones like estrogen that are responsible for forging female organs like vagina, uterus, breasts, and so on; the reason this does not happen in males is that the action of hormones like testosterone somehow prevents it.

Are female characteristics of body form and function, then, the only differences between males and females? Many of the more vociferous proponents of equality between men and women would have us believe so. The fact that girls prefer to play with dolls, and boys with cars, they say, arises not from their genes but from the environmental effect of their parents, who give them these toys according to their sex. Likewise differences in upbringing are responsible for other psychological differences between men and women, such as the capacity to recognize social problems and to interact accordingly (better in women), or the tendency toward depression (more common in women) or alcoholism (more common in men). In other words, these characteristics are presumed to be shaped by the environment, not by the genes. Is there really no genetic basis for behavioral differences between men and women? One possible difference has recently been highlighted, as follows. Women inherit one X chromosome from their father and one from their mother; men inherit their X chromosome only from their mother. If there were differences between maternal and paternal X chromosomes, differences that evolved over hundreds of thousands of years, could these not account for subtle differences in behavior between men and women? Some recent studies on the social skills of women with Turner's syndrome (in which women have only one X chromosome) suggest that those whose X chromosome is paternal do better than those whose X chromosome is maternal. Of course these are only very preliminary studies, and we need to wait until it becomes possible to screen all of the genes on the X chromosome and to compare the results for paternal and maternal X chromosomes, before reaching conclusions about a genetic basis for female behavior. That time is not so far away.

If one of the genes on the X chromosome carries a lethal mutation so that no functional protein is produced, the situation is much worse for males than for females. Take the case of hemophilia, namely, failure to produce factor VIII for blood clotting. The hereditary nature of this disease has long been recognized; it was prevalent in the royal families of Europe (Figure 40), and the young tsarevitch (son of Tsar Nicholas II) might well have died of the disease, had he not been shot in Ekaterinburg (now Sverdlovsk) in 1918 with the rest of his family. The gene for factor VIII is located on the X chromosome: males therefore make no factor VIII at all, but females will produce half the normal amount, which is sufficient for most situations (the mutation is recessive). This is because X chromosome inactivation is random: 50% of the cells in a tissue—liver in this case—will therefore have the healthy gene inactivated and produce no factor VIII; but the other 50% of cells will have the mutant gene inactivated and produce factor VIII as normal. Only in females who have inherited a nonfunctional gene from both parents, which is a much rarer event, is hemophilia as severe a disease as it is in males.

It should be mentioned here that our cells contain some DNA that is not part of our chromosomes. That DNA exists within the mitochondria, which are, as has been described, the powerhouse by which the energy derived from the oxidation of food is used for the synthesis of ATP. Some of the enzymes involved in those reactions are coded for use not on chromosomal genes, but on the genes of mitochondrial DNA, which is a single molecule about a 250th, or 0.4%, of the size of DNA in the smallest of our chromosomes. Unlike chromosomal DNA, most mitochondrial DNA is genetic, coding for proteins involved in oxidation and ATP synthesis; the rest codes for mitochondrial RNA. Scientists speculate that mitochondria represent the remains of symbiotic bacteria that infected the earliest living cells of animals and gave them the ability to synthesize ATP by the mechanism described in the previous chapter. That is as may be. What is relevant to this discussion of heredity is the fact that mitochondrial DNA is handed on only

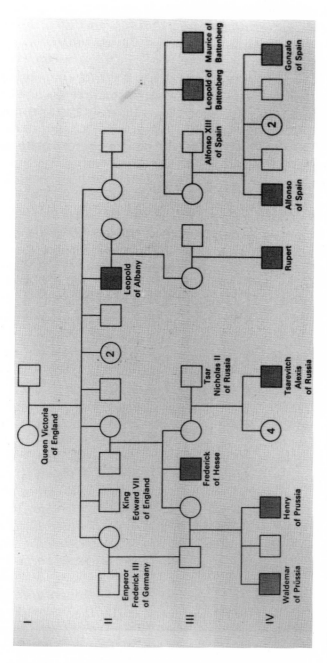

40. Inheritance of genes. Pedigree of hemophilia in the royal families of Europe. Females are symbolized by circles, normal males by open squares, hemophilic males by shaded squares. The Tsarevitch Alexis of Russia was the first male heir born to a reigning Russian tsar since the seventeenth century. From *Biochemistry* (first edition) by L. Stryer, 1975. Used with permission of W. H. Freeman & Company.

through females: The part of the sperm that enters an egg cell to fertilize it contains no mitochondria. The mitochondria of the fertilized egg, which reproduce themselves during subsequent cell divisions, are solely of maternal origin. Since the genes they contain are concerned only with energy metabolism, they are not particularly interesting so far as male versus female characteristics are concerned. What is much more important is that by analyzing mitochondrial DNA, one can track ancestries much more easily than through chromosomal DNA, which is a mixture of maternal and paternal DNA. If one were able to isolate Y chromosomes as a matter of routine—which is not at present the case—one would be able to trace purely paternal DNA, but there would be gaps every time a father failed to produce a male offspring. Analyzing mitochondrial DNA has helped to confirm the origin of several island populations in the Pacific Ocean and, more importantly, has led us to the conclusion that all races of man are rather closely related (see Figure 32 on p. 101).

In no area has interest in the relative contribution of genes versus the environment been expressed more keenly than in that relating to IQ, the "intelligence quotient." The debate as to nature versus nurture began over 100 years ago and it is raging still. At that time Francis Galton (Figure 41) in England suggested that one's mental capacity, like one's physical features, is inherited. He defined genius as "an ability that is exceptionally high, and at the same time inborn." The nature of inheritance, in terms of proteins that define our features and the processes that go on in our bodies, had to wait another 40 years before a link was made. It was another Englishman, Archibald Garrod, who coined the term "inborn errors of metabolism" to explain rare, inherited (i.e., inborn) diseases like alkaptonuria. Garrod noted that the urine of people with alkaptonuria turned black on standing. The reason for this was that a compound that he identified as homogentisic acid is excreted, and homogentisic acid turns black on being exposed to air. Subsequently a similar disease called phenylketonuria was found to be caused by the excretion of phenylketone. Both diseases are relatively rare single-gene disorders. Phenylketonuria, for example, occurs with an overall frequency of 1 in 10,000 live births; in Celtic populations the figure

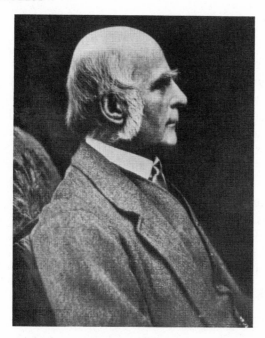

41. Francis Galton. Courtesy of The Wellcome Institute Library, London.

is five times higher. More common single gene disorders include cystic fibrosis, polycystic kidney disease (which accounts for some 10% of all kidney disease), and familial hypercholesterolemia (characterized by high cholesterol in the bloodstream). Garrod's hypothesis was that people with alkaptonuria excrete homogentisic acid because of an error in their metabolism. Recall that at that time the word enzyme had not been coined, nor its identity as protein realized; proteins had not even been purified sufficiently to appreciate that they have a fixed composition—this did not happen until the 1950s—and the molecular nature of inheritance was a mystery. We now know that Garrod was correct: Excretion of homogentisic acid and of phenylketone are consequences of the lack of a particular enzyme required for the metabolism of phenylalanine, one of the 20 amino acids found in proteins, as mentioned earlier. If the metabolism of our food is inborn, why not the workings of our mind? At the time that Francis Galton proposed a hereditary basis of intellect, of course, the link between metabolism and heredity had not yet been made. He was certainly a man before his time; so, for that matter, was Archibald Garrod. (Galton also coined the word eugenics to describe studies on people with "good" genes, the implication being that one should try to outbreed "bad" genes with "good." The consequences of such ideas in our own century have been less than happy.) At the time that Galton proposed a link between intelligence and heredity, this did not cause the stir that has subsequently flared up every time the quality of IQ in certain racial groups has been questioned. In 1869 Europeans and their descendants in the United States had little doubt of their intellectual superiority and were not too concerned whether it resulted from their forebears or their diet. They were, in any case, still reeling from the pronouncements of Thomas Huxley, champion of the views of the shy Charles Darwin, that man shares a common ancestry with the great apes.

Current research on IQ indicates that 50–70% is inherited, with the rest being attributed to the environment. It is environmental factors like diet, a cultured society, and so on, that probably account for the emergence of "clever" people at different times, in different places, though it must be stressed here that cleverness, intuition, or inventiveness are not the same as IQ. Where did such intellectual advances occur? In Babylon, China, India, Egypt, and Greece between 6000 and 2000 years ago, in the lands of the Arabs 1000 years ago, and—quite independently of all other civilizations—in Central America 1000 years ago. (The cleverness of the most advanced of these people, the Mayans who lived in what is now the Yucatan peninsula of Mexico and Guatemala, was limited. Although they had a very sophisticated mathematical system—based on the number 20—and excellent astronomy, they failed to appreciate the potential use of the wheel: They possessed these round objects, but only on children's toys.) Of all of these bursts of intellectual prowess, none has had greater impact on our life today than the development of the concept of zero. Quite apart from the philosophical significance of "nothing," Arabic numerals—in effect the decimal system—have revolutionized all aspects of mathematics and have made the development of computers possible. If you thought the Romans clever, try dividing CDXVIII by VIII in your head without recourse to Arabic numerals (168 by 8). The place where this break-through occurred was not the Arabian peninsula, but Gujarat in India, toward the end of the sixth century, and the numerical system became known as Arabic only because the Arabs invaded India shortly thereafter. Indians can also claim the invention of the game of chess. It began on a board of 64 squares, as used today, and contained pieces corresponding to a king and the corps of the ancient Indian army: elephant, horse, chariot or ship, and four footmen. At that time it was played with dice by four people, so the total number of pieces on the board was 32, the same number as today. The game was learned by the Persians, and when they were conquered by the Arabs it spread through the Middle East and into Spain. The Arabs dropped the dice, which had been used also by the Indians for gambling, since gambling is forbidden by the Koran, and the game began to be played by just two people, representing opposing armies. It was the Crusaders coming from Western Europe in the Middle Ages who substituted one of the pieces with the queen. The development of the game of chess is a good illustration of the blending of cultures that has occurred throughout the history of the Old World, and there has been contact, through traders as much as through warriors, between Western Europe, the Middle East, India, and China for over 2000 years. In contrast, the people of Mongolian descent who crossed the Bering Straits into North America prior to that time brought little of culture with them. Life in the frozen north was tough and their intellectual abilities were concentrated on sheer survival. Only after they had wandered down to the more equable climate of central and southern America did their cultures—the Mayans of Yucatan and Guatemala, the Aztecs of central Mexico, and the Incas of Peru—flourish.

Why do great civilizations decline? Often, of course, it is the result of being overrun by warring invaders, as happened to the American pre-Columbian peoples north and south of the equator. Sometimes there are other reasons. The great Arab (Islamic) tradition gradually declined after many centuries of glory probably because of religious fundamentalism; this had not played a major part during the time when the arts and sciences of Baghdad and Damascus, Cairo and Córdoba, were ruling the world.

Fundamentalism is incompatible with innovative thinking. There was little of it in Spain either, during the time of the Inquisition in the sixteenth century. To say that Arabs or Chinese, Indians or Greeks—or those of European descent in general—are more clever than American Indians or American Africans is quite unwarranted. To make such comparisons requires that the ground rules are the same; and growing up on an arid reservation in Idaho or in a slum in Harlem is not the same as growing up in Princeton or Southampton, Long Island. The importance of the right background for the emergence of clever ideas is one that is being addressed by the Nobel Foundation in Stockholm. It is planning a Centennial Exhibition in 2001 to commemorate 100 years of Nobel Prizes. The theme will be *The Culture of Creativity: Individuals and Milieus,* and the exhibition will pose the question of whether it is the process of individual creativity, or the existence of a creative milieu, that is the more important (in the arts and sciences).

The current view that IQ is 50–70% inherited is based very much on countless studies of twins, both identical and nonidentical. Identical twins occur when, for some reason, a fertilized egg splits in two at a very early stage and both halves survive to become separate fetuses; the genes of identical twins are therefore identical and any differences in looks or behavior can be regarded as environmental influences. Nonidentical twins occur when a female releases two or more eggs, instead of one, into the uterine tube—an occurrence that is fairly common with women on fertility drugs. In this case each egg is fertilized by a different sperm, and the genes of such twins are no more similar than the genes of siblings born of the same parents many years apart. I will not elaborate on the findings of the many studies that have been carried out. As might be anticipated, one group finds one degree of linkage between IQ and heredity, another finds something else. That is the trouble with measuring parameters as vague as IQ. Most, however, agree that identical twins separated at birth and brought up in different social backgrounds have similar IQs. This means that if we look hard enough at the DNA of clever people we should begin to find *some* genes that correlate with high IQ. Recent experiments by Richard Plomin at the Institute of Psychiatry in London, working with colleagues in the United States, appear to have done just that. They found that a particular variant of a gene (that codes for the cell surface receptor for an insulinlike growth factor) is twice as common in children of high IQ (mean of 136) as in children of average IQ (mean of 103). Of course it should be emphasized that correlation is not the same as cause. People who have fair hair may correlate with people who tend to get more severe sunburns, but that does not mean that having fair hair causes sunburn. It merely means that having fair hair and being susceptible to sunburn may have a common cause.

One study, carried out in Sweden, warrants description because it illustrates an important point. Identical and nonidentical twins over age 80 were compared for mental and verbal ability: Identical twins were much more alike than nonidentical twins, confirming earlier studies in four countries that had shown consistently greater correlations for identical twins than for nonidentical twins, at various ages from childhood to adulthood. What these results therefore indicate, in addition to confirming a strong genetic element, is that IQ does not change with age. This is surprising to those who think that environmental influences— learning from one's mistakes in life and so on—would increase a person's IQ with time. If this is not the case, then when *do* environmental influences play a role? (If they play no role at all, then the figure of 50–70% link with heredity should be 100%.) The answer is probably related to the fact that the brain cells develop already in late pregnancy and in the earliest years of life. After that there is not much change. Brain cells do not divide and grow like liver cells: Damage to brain cells is irreversible. It has already been noted that one of the consequences of severe malnutrition in children is mental retardation. This, too, is not reversed by diet. In short, whatever environmental effects like diet or an infectious episode have on our intelligence, they occur very early on, already before birth and for only a few years thereafter, during the time that the myriad of brain cells and their connections are being laid down. From then on, we are programmed to be as clever or as stupid for the rest of our lives. Of course this does not mean that we do not learn new ideas, languages, or physical skills during the rest of our lives: It is whether we learn them well or badly, whether we remember them well or badly, that is determined at an early age. A final point. Since the molecular details of the way that environmental influences shape IQ in early life are not known, we cannot say whether they act on genes in the way that environmental influences—like viruses, ionizing radiations, or diet—act on genes that are associated with the progression toward cancer. They are as likely to do so as not. In that case—as with cancer or any other disease—the distinction is not between genes and the environment, but between *inherited* genes and the environment.

From what has been said so far, it is clear that a complete analysis of the genes of an individual should tell us a great deal about that person's susceptibility to develop particular diseases during his or her lifetime. The day that such information will be available is upon us. However, we must remember that many common diseases will turn out to be multigenic: that is to say, more than one gene contributes to the onset of the disease. Some types of cancer, for example, arise if any one or more of 5–10 different proteins—i.e., 5–10 different gene products—is faulty. We have long known that the progression to cancer is a multistep process, controlled by specific proteins that are now coming to be identified. This is in contrast to diseases like sickle-cell anemia or G-6-PD deficiency, where a defect in only one gene explains the condition. Even in such cases, however, other genes may play secondary roles in promoting or ameliorating the disease, in the way that environmental factors like nutrition or a microbial infection do.

If frank diseases like cancer or heart disease are multigenic, then it is even more likely that traits like homosexuality, criminal behavior, or intelligence will prove to be so: Reports that "the gene" for homosexuality, criminal behavior, or intelligence has been discovered should be treated with extreme skepticism. Moreover, as is emphasized throughout this book, our genes are only a part of the answer: Our relationship with the environment plays an equally important part. Also, as will become apparent in a later chapter, many of the thought processes in our brains probably depend as much on *modification* of proteins—through "second messenger" events like phosphorylation of proteins—as on genetically determined *synthesis* of proteins.

By the year 2005 the Human Genome Project, a multinational endeavor that aims to sequence every chromosome in its entirety, should be completed. One should then be able to analyze any gene at will and see whether it is faulty or not. This, of course, presupposes that the chromosomes that have been sequenced all come from individuals who are healthy at every point, which is unlikely even if we could recognize a healthy gene when we see one. Moreover the sequencing is being done not on the DNA of one or two individuals, but on that of several different people (using the DNA from sperm and from a number of cell lines of human tissue growing in sterile cultures). At present we know only about 50% of the genes in our chromosomes. Then there is the difficulty of knowing what any gene actually does: Reading the nucleotide sequence of a gene allows one to predict the amino acid sequence of the relevant protein, but this is not the same as knowing its function. On the other hand, the knowledge that has already been gained from sequencing the chromosomes that make up the genome of the yeast *Saccharomyces cerevisiae,* as well as the single chromosomes of several bacteria, will help to identify many genes by analogy. In addition, knowledge of the genome of such infectious microbes as *Haemophilus influenzae* or *Helicobacter pylori,* will aid in better design of antibiotics and vaccines with which to curb their ill effects: To know your enemy well is the first requirement in defeating him.

What difference will it actually make to our lives to know that we have certain mutations in our genes that make a heart attack or the onset of cancer more likely? Should we not refrain from smoking, overeating, and underexercising anyway? And is not the knowledge of an impending disease likely to cause us so much stress that we are in danger of incurring the disease through this factor alone? True, knowledge of our genes may be accompanied by the availability of so many new drugs to keep unwanted ailments at bay that we may not need to worry, but this is an unlikely scenario. Unfortunately, discovery of new diseases has not been matched by discovery of new therapies. HIV infection leading to AIDS is a prime example. The disease was recognized as being caused by an infectious microbe, the virus HIV, in the mid-1980s; within a matter of years the molecular structure of the virus was identified and its entire genome sequenced. It seemed only a matter of time before a successful drug or vaccine would be developed. Ten years on, and we are still waiting. Insofar as bacterial infections are concerned, no new class of antibiotic has been discovered for thirty years.

In some cases there is no doubt that the new knowledge of our genetic makeup will be of immense benefit. Knowing that one's gene for absorbing an essential nutrient like folic acid is faulty, for example, allows one to rectify the deficiency by ingesting extra folic acid before pernicious anemia sets in. In any case, will we not be able to rectify faulty genes by replacing them? So far, the results of gene therapy have not been particularly encouraging, but then the technique is still in its infancy. No one at present is contemplating replacing the genes in our germ cells, which we would pass on to the next generation; replacing or otherwise modifying the genes outside our germ cells for medical reasons is, in principle, no different than modifying the levels of insulin in our veins by injecting the hormone, or increasing our content of factor VIII. Perhaps then, provided we have no major health problems, we should just continue to sit in our armchairs, read the scientific journals and newspapers about startling new discoveries, smile at it all, and go for a walk to buy vegetables and fresh fruit.

However, there will be instances when we shall be unable to take so relaxed a view. We may wish to buy a new house or an automobile, open a bank account, or take out a new credit card. We may need to apply for a new job or move to another country. Will the relevant authority—insurance company, bank manager, prospective employer, immigration official—not require us to have a complete DNA screen first, and if they do not like the results, charge us more or deny our request outright? These are considerations we will not be able to escape. In order to prevent them becoming a nightmare, we need to resort to the measures available in a democracy for curbing unwarranted power and interference in our lives. But in order to make our case, we need to be well informed. We need to understand the molecules within us.

———————————➤◆◄———————————

This chapter has examined the causes of disease, in particular the relationship between genetic factors and environmental ones. These turn out to overlap, in the sense that some environmental factors affect our genes. But the distinction between what we inherit, and to what we expose ourselves, remains.

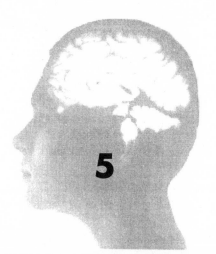

5

MICROBIAL INFECTIONS AND
THE IMMUNE SYSTEM

ntil a few hundred years ago, when sanitary conditions began to improve dramatically and hygiene became a way of life, most people died of a microbial infection. The death rate among babies and infants was particularly high. Even today, death from an infection is second only to heart disease world-wide. And infections from which we recover are the most prevalent causes of mild disease: indispositions such as a head cold or a stomach upset. More working days are lost as a result of an infection like influenza than from any other cause. What are microbes, and how can we fight against them? First we should say that we are concerned here only with infectious microbes, those that get inside our bodies and cause disease. The great majority of microbes do not do this—they are nonpathogenic to humans—in just the way that most animals pose no threat to us either. The word microbe implies that they are small (*mikros* is Greek for "small"), but just how small is small?

The size of microbes that infect us varies enormously (Figure 42). A tapeworm (containing many thousands of cells) can be more than 1 yard (1 meter) long, though it is less than a thousandth of

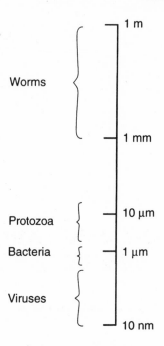

42. Infectious organisms. Their sizes vary from a meter (a yard) in the case of a tapeworm to a hundred millionth of that in the case of the smallest viruses.

this size when it enters with our food. The smallest viruses are some 10 nanometers (a two hundred and fifty-thousandth of an inch) in size. Protozoa and bacteria are of intermediate sizes; our cells, for comparison, are similar in size to the largest protozoa.

Infectious microbes overcome our body's natural protection against them and gain entry in one of five ways: in food and drink through the mouth; in infected air through the nose; through the skin via the bite of an infected insect or other animal; through sexual intercourse with infected partners; and less commonly, through being born of an infectious mother. The type of disease to which we succumb generally reflects the mode of entry. Respiratory viruses like influenza, for example, do not survive at the temperature of our bloodstream (37°C or 98°F) and multiply only in our nasal passages where the temperature is lower. A runny nose is the direct result of such an infection. The fever, headache, joint ache, and so on occur because the cells in which the virus multiplies trigger the release of molecules, such as certain proteins called cytokines. It is cytokines acting on tissues far away from the initial site of an infection that cause many symptoms of microbial disease. For this reason, and because quite different microbes are capable of invading a particular organ like lung, intestine, or liver, it is important to identify the rogue agent. Respiratory diseases may be caused by bacteria like streptococci or pneumococci, or they may be caused by viruses like influenza, whooping cough, or the common cold virus; stomach upsets and diarrhea may be caused by protozoa like *Entamoeba histolytica*, by bacteria like *Salmonella, Escherichia coli,* or *Vibrio cholerae,* or by rotaviruses; hepatitis may be caused by *Entamoeba hystolytica* or by different types of hepatitis virus. It is no use treating viral infections with antibiotics, for example, because viruses are not sensitive to their action.

How prevalent are different microbial infections? Overall, a third of deaths worldwide are caused by a microbial infection; that is, approximately 17 million out of a total of 52 million deaths per year. The remainder result, predominantly, from heart disease and cancer. Of those 17 million deaths from microbes, acute respiratory infections are the biggest killer (4.4 million), followed by tuberculosis and diarrheal diseases (each 3.1 million), malaria (2.1 million), and hepatitis B (the form of the hepatitis virus that is particularly prevalent in China and Southeast Asia: 1.1 million). AIDS, measles, and other diseases caused by viruses (whooping cough), bacteria (neonatal tetanus), and worms (roundworm and hookworm) make up the rest. Of course these diseases are not spread evenly around the world; deaths from microbial infections are much lower in the developed countries of the Far East, Europe, and North America than in the rest of the world; we saw in the last chapter that AIDS, for example, is rising particularly rapidly in Africa. Partly these differences reflect geographical factors; the developed countries of the northern hemisphere are some way distant from equatorial and subequatorial regions where malaria, for example, is rife; this was not always so. Until the 1920s malaria (from the Italian *mala aria*—bad air—of the marshes in which the mosquitoes that carry it live) was present in southern Europe and if global warming continues it may return. Other reasons are also fairly obvious: better sanitary conditions (since many infectious diseases are spread through poor hygiene), better nutrition (since a malnourished body cannot combat an infection as well as a healthy one), and the use of vaccines and antibiotics (to which most of the population in the underdeveloped world does not have access because of poverty). How do vaccines and antibiotics work?

Much has been made of the similarity in molecular composition and structure between microbes and higher organisms, namely, plants and animals. Each consists of protein, carbohydrate, fat, and nucleic acids, and these molecules function in similar ways. Yet there are also obvious differences between microbes on the one hand, and plants and animals on the other. For one thing, most microbes are single-celled organisms. They lack the special structures like skin or shell that protects animals from the environment. Instead, bacteria—and the present discussion will focus on bacteria because they cause the majority of microbial diseases—have developed special molecules for protection that are not found in animals. These molecules make up a barrier or wall on the outside of the membrane (the plasma membrane, which is similar to that in animals) that surrounds the contents of each bacterium. In some species of bacterium, like *Salmonella, Escherichia coli, Helicobacter,* or *Vibrio cholerae,* the protective layer, or cell wall, is made up of fat and carbohydrate (known as lipopolysaccharide); in others, like streptococci, staphylococci, or bacilli, it is made up of a meshwork of amino acids and carbohydrate (known as peptidoglycan). Cell walls are not found in animals, so interference with their synthesis or function is unlikely to affect animal cells; that is, the toxicity in animal cells—and we are concerned here particularly with human cells—of molecules that inhibit the function of bacterial cell walls, is low. This is precisely how penicillin works to destroy bacteria. The word antibiotic was originally coined to describe the properties of a molecule that is made and secreted by one type of microbe, for example the mold *Penicillium,* that kills other microbes, for example bacteria like staphylococci; although molds also have cell walls, they are different from bacterial ones. Nowadays the term is used for chemically synthesized molecules, like derivatives of penicillin, too.

Antibiotics against the cell wall (the lipopolysaccharide coating) of bacteria like *Salmonella* have not so far been found. On the other hand, the molecular structure of bacterial lipopolysaccharide is sufficiently different from any human molecule to make it a good candidate for a vaccine; vaccines, as will be described below, are molecules not found in our bodies that cause the destruction of microbes (vaccines directed against cancer cells are also now being developed). Other targets for antibiotic action against bacteria, like *Mycobacterium tuberculosis*, the causative agent of TB, however, exist. The reason is as follows. Although the synthesis of protein in bacteria is in general very similar to that in man, it is not identical. The similarity lies in the fact that in each case specific genes (stretches of DNA) code for specific proteins. In each case a stretch of DNA is copied into a molecule of RNA. In each case the sequence of nucleotides (A, G, C, and U) in that RNA is then "read off" and translated into a protein; every three nucleotides in the RNA code for a specific amino acid in the protein. In each case translation of RNA into protein involves several other molecules: two types of RNA (called transfer RNA and ribosomal RNA) and a number of protein molecules, some of which act as enzymes to make the whole process go. Although similar in function, the precise structures of the RNA and protein molecules are different in bacteria and man. Different enough so that antibiotics secreted by *Streptomyces* (a mold similar to *Penicillium*), like streptomycin, gentamycin, or neomycin, inhibit protein synthesis—and therefore growth—of several types of bacterium without an effect on protein synthesis in humans; an early use of streptomycin, half a century ago, was against tuberculosis. The use of antibiotics of this group has, over the subsequent years, declined. This is partly because they exert quite a number of toxic side effects, but mainly because most strains of bacterium that infect humans are now resistant to their action.

Bacterial resistance to antibiotics is now so widespread that there is a serious danger of not being able to treat the next case of pneumonia or blood poisoning with an antibiotic at all. Indeed that situation has already arisen in Japan, where a patient recently proved to be resistant to every single antibiotic that was tried. How does resistance come about? It is because bacteria divide much more rapidly than animal cells—every hour or so, compared with a day or more in the most rapidly dividing cells like certain white cells or the cells lining the intestine. Mutations are therefore generated much more frequently than is the case in humans. Many mutations will either have no effect or they will be deleterious, but some will result in a gene being expressed in much greater an amount—thousands of times more—than before. If such a bacterial gene codes, for example, for an enzyme that is able to break down a particular antibiotic so that it is no longer toxic to the bacterium, that bacterium will survive. Those bacteria, the mutant ones that possess the antibiotic-degrading enzyme, will then rapidly outgrow the parent bacteria that are killed by the presence of the antibiotic.

This is exactly what can happen to bacterial populations inside the body of someone taking an antibiotic. That is why it is important to follow the instructions on a prescription rigorously: The antibiotic should be taken for long enough to kill most of the bacteria so that there are insufficient survivors left to rekindle the infection. However, it should not be taken for so long that resistant strains begin to emerge. Should there be evidence that this is occurring, one should ask one's doctor to quickly switch to another antibiotic that cannot be degraded by the resistant strain. All of this presupposes that one is able to continuously monitor how many bacteria are left, and whether they are resistant to the antibiotic one is taking: a pretty tall order for someone taking an antibiotic like penicillin for a mild infection! Every problem stimulates solutions, and pharmaceutical companies are frantically trying to synthesize derivatives of the limited number of antibiotics in existence that are insensitive to the enzymes of mutant bacteria. But—you guessed it—once the chemically modified antibiotics are used extensively, strains resistant to *them* begin to emerge. It would not be an overstatement to say that the prognosis for dealing with resistant bacteria is not good.

If the situation with regard to bacterial infections seems gloomy, that for viral infections could hardly be worse. In this instance the problem is twofold. First, there are very few drugs against viral infections at all. Contrary to public opinion, antibiotics should never be used to fight viruses because they are unaffected by them. Worse, any bacteria lurking in our bodies—too few to generate an infection—might be affected, insofar as the presence of the antibiotic would encourage the growth of a resistant strain; then next time conditions favor bacterial growth, the strains that emerge will be accompanied by antibiotic-resistant ones. Physicians do sometimes prescribe antibiotics if they are not sure whether the infection is a bacterial or a viral one, on the assumption that it can't do any harm, and even if the infection *is* a viral one, the antibiotic will prevent a secondary—bacterial—infection in a body weakened by the virus. The danger inherent in this line of argument has been stressed. The second problem is that viruses, like bacteria, generate mutant forms. The reason why it has proved so difficult to find drugs against viruses is that they live and multiply inside the cells of a host—be it a bacterium, plant, or animal. Viruses enter one of our cells by binding to some molecule on the cell surface whose function is something quite different; it just so happens that a part of the virus resembles the molecular structure of whatever is supposed to bind the receptor on the cell surface, like a hormone, a neurotransmitter, a cytokine, or some other molecule. It is like counterfeit money: not exactly the same as the real thing, but sufficiently close to fool a shop assistant or cab driver. Because molecules bound at the cell surface tend eventually to be internalized, virus particles are treated in the same way by a cell fooled by them (Figure 43). Once inside the cell, the virus particle opens up and releases its nucleic acid (DNA or RNA). This is where the trouble starts. For now the virus uses the machinery of the cell to make 100 or more new copies of itself, all of which then burst out of the cell and infect 100 more cells. Sometimes the virus bides its time. The chickenpox virus (a member of the herpes family), for example, infects young children, causing the characteristic symptoms of spots in the skin. The disease is generally not serious and soon dies down. But in some individuals the virus remains in the body—in nerve cells—for years on end. It is not replicated, and therefore does not set up an infection. Suddenly the virus breaks loose and starts to divide. It now causes shingles, a very irritating, and sometimes extremely

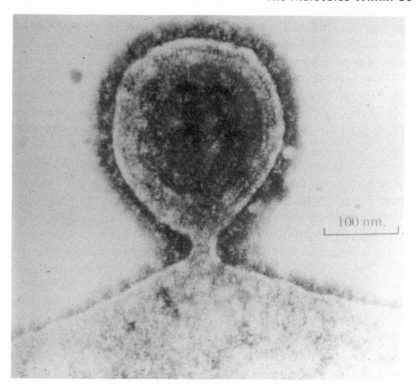

43. A virus entering a cell. Electron micrograph of a paramyxovirus (Sendai virus; the same group as mumps, measles, and rubella virus) invading a cell by fusion of its membrane with that of the cell. The dark material outside the light phospholipid membrane of virus and cell is made of proteins similar to the H and N proteins of influenza virus (a close relative). The dark material in the center of the virus consists of other proteins and of RNA (the genetic material of viruses like measles, mumps, rubella, or influenza). Taken by Dr. Stuart Knutton in the author's laboratory and reproduced with Dr. Knutton's permission.

painful, disease. Patients are generally treated with drugs against the pain (known as postherpetic neuralgia). Very few drugs can successfully fight against the herpesvirus itself, and even fewer can combat other equally common viruses.

The reason for our inability to fight viruses is that there is so little to attack. Unlike bacteria they have no special molecules associated with them. Outside the body they are inert particles consisting of protein and DNA or RNA, sometimes surrounded by a membrane similar to that of our cells—indeed derived from our cells following an infection. Inside our cells the viral molecules are too like our own DNA, RNA, or protein to make them suitable targets, and the enzymes they use for replicating their DNA or RNA and protein are mostly ours anyway. What enzymes of its own that a virus does introduce into the cell have naturally been the focus for the synthesis of appropriate drugs, and some limited success with drugs like acyclovir, which interfere with nucleic acid synthesis, has been achieved with herpesviruses. A related drug—AZT or zidovudine—seemed at first to be effective against HIV, but after more carefully controlled clinical trials enthusiasm for it waned. It may, however, be of use in combination with other treatments. One of these is based on inhibitors of a viral protease. Viruses like HIV make their own protease (an enzyme that splits proteins), which is required for the assembly of new infectious virus particles. Because the protease of HIV is slightly different from the proteases found in our cells, there has been much activity in trying to design drugs that bind selectively to the HIV protease. Some of these have now come on to the market. Overall, however, we have few cures for viral infections. How, in the face of this unsatisfactory situation, have we been able to improve our survival rate—especially that of young children—over the last 100 years or so? Through vaccines, which boost our immune system.

The human body is protected against microbial attack in a number of ways. The skin prevents most microbes from entering our bodies by this route, especially as sweat contains some antimicrobial molecules. Only if the skin is actually ruptured, as occurs when an insect such as a fly bites us, can microbes—present in the saliva of the fly—penetrate the skin. This is the way the malarial parasite gains access to our bloodstream. Microbes that enter by mouth or nose become enmeshed in sticky mucus that is secreted and is eventually swallowed. However, it is clear that many microbes do gain access through mouth or nose: Bacteria like *Salmonella* or *Vibrio cholerae* and viruses like rotaviruses, which enter via the mouth, are common causes of food poisoning and other gastrointestinal diseases; bacteria like streptococci and viruses like influenza and rhinovirus (the common cold virus), which enter via the nose, are common causes of respiratory diseases. Before such microbes can initiate an infection, however, they have to overcome another line of defense: the immune system.

Animals began to develop an immune system millions of years ago. First it was a nonspecific defense mechanism—present in primitive worms onwards—against anything foreign that enters the body, which we still retain today. Then it developed into a highly specific system—around the time that early forms of fish evolved—that is capable of recognizing one particular molecular structure out of millions of others, and subsequently destroying all foreign bodies that display that structure. The major players involved in the immune system, both nonspecific and specific, are the white cells of the blood. Like the red cells, they are derived ultimately from the bone marrow (Figure 44). White cells are divided into leukocytes and lymphocytes. The main function of leukocytes is to destroy foreign substances such as bacteria, protozoa (single-celled organisms like the malarial parasite), and metazoa (many-celled organisms like tapeworms); viruses are destroyed largely by lymphocytes. The main type of leukocyte, also called a phagocyte (from the Greek for "a cell that eats"), ingests anything that sticks to its surface—be it a piece of dust or a bacterium (Figure 45). Phagocytes circulating in the bloodstream are called neutrophils; phagocytes that are present inside tissues are called macrophages. Once the foreign particle has been internalized by the phagocytes, the offending molecules are degraded by powerful enzymes that are not found in any of the other cells of the body. This is nonspecific immunity. It is made specific, and more powerful, through the mechanisms of specific immunity that involve the lymphocytes.

There are two classes of lymphocyte, called B and T cells. It is with the B cells that we are concerned for the moment. B cells display on their surface a protein called an immunoglobulin or antibody. Immunoglobulins are a family of 100 million members, each immunoglobulin molecule being very slightly different from all others. The origin of this diversity is not that there are 100 million immunoglobulin genes; there are actually relatively few. Diversity is created by the fact that an immunoglobulin molecule

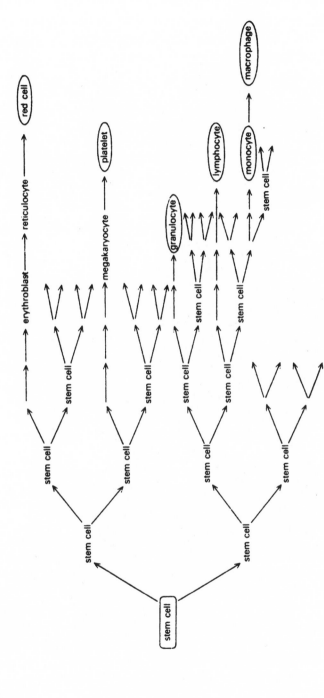

44. Blood cells. The maturation of red cells, platelets, and white cells from common precursor cells takes place in the bone marrow. From *An Introduction to Human Biochemistry* by C. A. Pasternak, Oxford University Press, 1979.

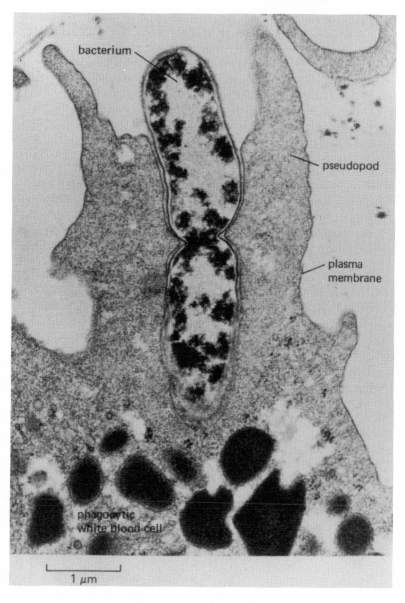

45. Phagocytosis. A phagocytic white blood cell is shown devouring a bacterium, which is caught in the process of dividing in two. From *The Molecular Biology of the Cell* (Fig. 6-80) by B. Alberts, D. Bray, J. Lewis, M. Raff, K. Roberts, and J. D. Watson, Garland Publishing Inc., 1983, with permission.

contains several segments, each of which is coded by a different gene. The part of an immunoglobulin molecule that is most different in each of the millions of immunoglobulin molecules (because of a different combination of amino acids) is appropriately called the variable (V) region of the molecule; the remainder is known as the constant (C) region (Figure 46). Each molecule actually consists of four separate chains of amino acids, held together by covalent (–S–S–) bonds, which were described in Chapter 2. There are two short chains—called *light* (L)—and two long chains—called *heavy* (H). Each chain has a variable region at one end, and a constant region at the other end. Between these two regions of a light chain is a separate, short region of amino acids called the *joining* (J) region. Between the V and H regions of a heavy chain, there are two separate, short regions (called D and J). When the light chain of an immunoglobulin molecule is being made, a V gene is selected from the different V genes on the chromosome, a J gene is selected, and a C gene is selected. In the case of the heavy chain of an immunoglobulin molecule, V, D, J, and C genes are selected. From each combination of gene segments, the respective protein chains—two light chains and two heavy chains—are made and assembled into complete immunoglobulin

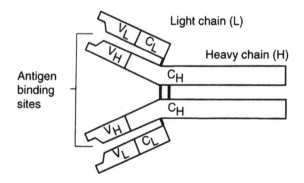

46. Immunoglobulins. All immunoglobulin types contain two light and two heavy chains. Each chain is made up of a variable (V) and a constant (C) region; the J and D regions are not shown, as they are very short in relation to the V and C regions. The site at which foreign molecules (antigens) bind to the variable regions of an immunoglobulin (also called an antibody) is indicated.

molecules. Imagine a hinged ladder of the sort that you stand on to prune your hedge or paint your ceiling (in other words not one that you have to lean against a wall). Now imagine that you are going to make such a ladder out of Lego™. The shorter, supporting, part of the ladder will be made out of 3 different pieces of Lego (called V, J, and C); it corresponds to a light chain. The longer part, which one climbs to reach the top, will be made out of 4 different pieces (called V, D, J, and C); it corresponds to a heavy chain. Now imagine that each piece, V, D, J, and C, comes in one of three different colors—say red, white, and blue. How many different ladders can you make? Assume that any color can combine with any other color. The answer is that you can make $3 \times 3 \times 3 = 27$ short parts of the ladder and $3 \times 3 \times 3 \times 3 = 81$ long parts of the ladder. Since any short part can combine with any long part, the total number of different ladders you can make is $27 \times 81 = 2187$. Note that this relatively large number of possibilities has been generated not by having a large number of different colors from which to choose—the number was only 3—but by having the ladder made up in separate segments, though again a small number—just 3 segments for the short part and 4 segments for the long part. This is precisely the way that diversity is created in immunoglobulins.

The number of segments that make up an immunoglobulin molecule is the same as in the example of the ladder, but the number of genes from which any one segment is made—corresponding to the three colors in the example of the ladder—is much greater. There are in fact 250–1000 different genes specifying the V region of heavy chains, and several hundreds of different genes specifying the V region of light chains (the exact numbers for humans are not yet known; we await the complete sequencing of the human genome). There are 10 different genes for the D region and 4 for the J region of heavy chains, and 4 different genes for the J region of light chains. Since, as with the example of the ladder, any one region can combine with any other region to make a full molecule, the total number of different molecules is 250–1000 × 10 × 4 (heavy chains) × several 100 × 4 (light chains), or around 100,000,000 different immunoglobulin molecules. Emphasis is on this way of creating diversity by shuffling a relatively small number of genes—2000 at most—rather than by having a very large number of genes—100 million genes for 100 million immunoglobulin molecules—because it is biologically more efficient. Recall that there are probably no more than 100,000 genes altogether in our chromosomes and that the total amount of DNA (the entire human genome) is only 10 times longer. In other words, the total amount of DNA in each of our cells is 1% of the amount that would be required just for immunoglobulin synthesis if each immunoglobulin were specified by a separate gene. This way of generating diversity is not limited to immunoglobulins. We shall see later that it is also the way that diversity is created in T lymphocytes. Moreover a similar mechanism is at work insofar as diversity in our looks and behavior is concerned: The subtle differences between parents and offspring are generated during the formation of egg and sperm, when different parts of two chromosomes are recombined to form one chromosome. In the case of immunoglobulins, the recombination event during which the different gene products, namely, the different segments that make up the protein chains, are selected and zipped together, occurs during the maturation of the immune system. That process begins in the fetus around the 10th week of pregnancy, lasts throughout childhood, and then begins to decline.

The structure of these amazing molecules—namely, immunoglobulins made by B lymphocytes—was unraveled by a brilliant piece of analytical chemistry carried out 30 years ago by two scientists working independently of each other: Gerald Edelman in the United States and Rodney Porter in England (Figure 47). Any one B cell has just one type of immunoglobulin (in hundreds of identical copies) displayed on its surface, so there are 100 million different types of B cell. When a foreign particle like a bacterium encounters a B lymphocyte whose immunoglobulin has just the right kind of complementary shape in its variable part—as a kind of groove or pocket, exactly like that in an enzyme—bacterium and B cell momentarily combine; the bacterium is referred to as an antigen, and the immunoglobulin on the B cell as an antibody. The act of interaction between the two triggers a response in the B cell. Imagine yourself in the vault of a bank;

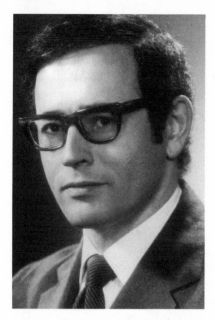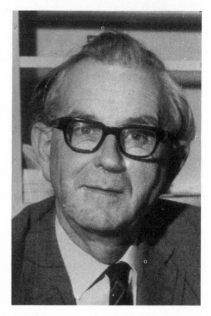

47. Gerald Edelman and Rodney Porter. Nobel laureates, 1972. Edelman (left) and Porter (right) worked out the structure of immunoglobulins independently of each other. Copyright (Edelman): The Nobel Foundation, Stockholm.

you are surrounded by hundreds of safe deposit boxes, and are holding a key. It will fit the lock of only one of those boxes. You try each lock in turn. Finally you find one that fits. A response is triggered: The box opens. In the case of a B cell the response is as follows: It now secretes immunoglobulin of exactly the same type as was on its surface originally. The secreted immunoglobulin molecules bind to any of the original bacteria that are still in the bloodstream. Bacteria with immunoglobulin bound to them are taken up and destroyed by phagocytes, just like bacteria without immunoglobulin on them. The difference is that recognition by phagocytes of bacteria is much better if the latter have immunoglobulin on them, and the process of gobbling them up and destroying them is also much improved. This, in essence, is the difference between the nonspecific and the specific immune response. In the nonspecific case, bacteria are rather inefficiently taken up and destroyed by phagocytes; in the specific case, the process is much more efficient because phagocytes destroy a bacterium–immunoglobulin complex better than they do a bacterium alone.

The story does not end here. First, there is an additional mechanism by which the immune system attacks particles like bacteria. This involves a group of proteins, called complement (they complement the mechanism described above), that are secreted by the liver and act in an enzymatic cascade rather like the blood clotting proteins. The trigger for their action is—like that for phagocytes—the presence of a complex between immunoglobulin and a foreign particle like a bacterium. The end result of the action of complement is that the proteins concerned form themselves into a hollow plug, like the drain of a wash basin. The plug then inserts itself into the membrane of the bacterium, forming a large hole. The contents of the bacterium now leak out and the bacterium is killed.

Complexes containing bacterium, immunoglobulin, and complement proteins are taken up and destroyed by phagocytes even more avidly than are complexes without complement proteins. The process could be called superspecific immunity. You may wonder why complement proteins do not form a plug that destroys our own cells. The answer is that immunoglobulins do not recognize any molecular features on the surface of our cells, and do not therefore bind to form a complex that would trigger the complement cascade. But if for some reason a molecule appears on one of our cells that is recognized as foreign, then it becomes subject to destruction by a complement. Such an attack of our cells by an overstimulated immune response leads to a condition called autoimmunity. This underlies diseases such as diabetes (destruction of insulin-producing cells of the pancreas), thyroid disease (destruction of thyroid cells), multiple sclerosis (destruction of nerves), and others as described below. The reasons for the display of a molecule on our cells that mimics a foreign one are not yet clear; they are often associated with a prior infection.

The second part of the story concerning bacterial destruction is as follows. After an initial bacterial–B cell contact leading to the secretion of immunoglobulin, the B cell divides to form "memory" cells, each of which displays the one immunoglobulin—out of the possible 100 million—that matched the bacterium. The next time this bacterium gains entry into the circulation, the memory cells begin to divide many times to form thousands of identical cells (a clone) all secreting the original immunoglobulin, which is now present in the bloodstream at more than a 100-fold higher concentration than was the case the first time around. Against such a massive response, the bacterium has little chance of survival. This is the way we become immune to bacterial infections (Figure 48). The essential role of the immune system in augmenting the action of phagocytes (the white cells that eat up bacteria and destroy them) has even found itself into the theater. In George Bernard Shaw's *The Doctors' Dilemma*, written over 90 years ago, Sir Colenso Ridgeon constantly advises his medical colleagues to "stimulate the phagocytes."

The mechanism by which an initial infection leads to the production of memory cells and a subsequent massive release of immunoglobulin is also the way that vaccines against bacteria work. A vaccine mimics the invading bacterium in initiating a primary immunoglobulin response and the production of memory cells, so that should the actual bacterium invade the body some time after the vaccination, it will be effectively destroyed. Vaccines may be made of heat-killed bacteria (to destroy their ability to infect), or of just a part of the bacterial surface—like a protein or a lipopolysaccharide—that is recognized by an appropriate immunoglobulin, and that is not in itself infectious. Because infection by a bacterium is often extremely unpleasant—and may even kill the host, especially if the latter is an infant or a young child (whose immune system is not fully developed) or an aged person (whose immune system is beginning to flag)—vaccination is what has saved countless lives against such bacterial infections as tuberculosis, diphtheria, typhoid, tetanus, and cholera. Vaccines against infectious viruses have also been produced, as will be described shortly. But it is impossible to predict how effective a vaccine will be: As yet we have no vaccine against malaria, leprosy, or many other serious microbial infections.

The immune system's response to viruses is somewhat different than that to bacteria. In this instance the T lymphocytes are involved. T lymphocytes are similar to B lymphocytes in having a molecule that resembles immunoglobulins displayed on their surface. Again, there are some 100 million different T cells, each displaying a slightly different type of molecule on its surface. These are produced—like immunoglobulins—from a relatively small number of genes coding for different regions of the molecule by recombination of genes during development of the immune system. The molecules recognize not free virus, but virus-infected cells. Recall that viruses live and multiply only inside cells. What part of the virus is recognized by the T cells? Not, as one might suppose (and many did suppose, until relatively recently), the outside of the virus as it is about to leave (or enter) the cell. What the T cells recognize is a small part of any one of the proteins that constitute the virus: a part that is only some 8–10 amino acids long (such short stretches of amino acids are called peptides). Protein-degrading enzymes, like the proteases discussed earlier, in cells that are infected with virus, degrade viral proteins at random to produce peptides. Of course, if the infection is particularly virulent, the cell may die before it has a chance to produce such virally derived peptides. As with all disease and our body's ability to counteract it, there is a fine line separating progression of disease and progression of recovery.

Recognition of viral peptides at the surface of infected cells is only part of the story. In order for the killer T cell to be triggered, it has to recognize the viral peptide in combination with a protein that is present on the surface of all cells. That protein is part of a family of proteins called major histocompatibility complex (MHC) or human leukocyte antigen (HLA). These proteins are also involved in the rejection of foreign tissue from the body following a tissue transplant, which is how they got their name. MHC proteins vary slightly from person to person, which is why an identical twin makes the best recipient for a transplant. For other transplants, even when derived from a close relative, it is necessary to minimize the immune response in order to prevent rejection of the transplant. Immunosuppressive drugs like cyclosporin work reasonably well, though rejection of transplants in the long term remains a major challenge for surgeons: One cannot keep suppressing the immune system for fear that the patient will succumb to a microbial infection.

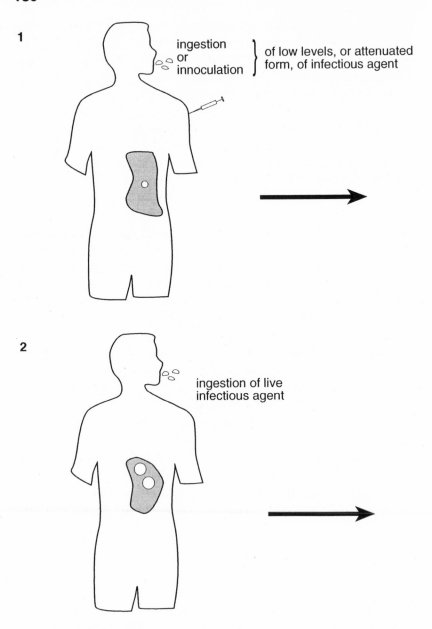

48. The immune response in protection. From *An Introduction to Human Biochemistry* by C. A. Pasternak, Oxford University Press, 1979.

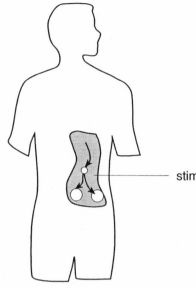

stimulation of lymphocytes

slight symptoms of disease

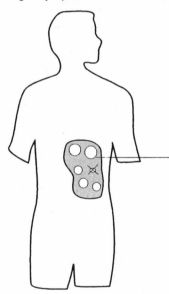

neutralization of infectious
agent by lymphocytes and
elimination of neutralized
agent by macrophages

48. (*continued*)

The combination of viral peptide—in a groove, as with immunoglobulins—and MHC protein (Figure 49) is then recognized by T cells. Two types of T cell play a part. The first is a cytotoxic or killer cell, a member of the T8 group of cells, that acts rather like activated complement: It punctures a hole in the plasma membrane of the virally infected cell (through proteins that are similar both in form and in function to those involved in attack by complement) and kills it. Killing one of our cells might be thought not to be very good therapy; but actually killing a few cells out of the billions that make up a functioning tissue is hardly noticed by the body. It is a lot better than allowing a nasty virus to multiply and infect a great many more cells.

The second type of T cell that is involved in immunity against viruses is one that gives rise to memory cells, just as with B cells. As a result, a second infection by the same virus is rapidly dealt with. As with B cells, this is the basis for making viral vaccines; again, intact, heat-killed (i.e., noninfectious) viruses, as well as viral proteins and viral peptides, have been used as vaccines. But, again, as with bacteria, success is not always assured. We have had great success with smallpox vaccine (to which we shall return in Chapter 7), and have just about eliminated the disease off the face of the earth. Other vaccines, like those against polio, yellow fever, measles, mumps, influenza, and several other viruses, have also proved effective. But we have no vaccine against HIV, herpes, and many other clinically important viruses.

The situation with regard to HIV is particularly serious since, as already mentioned, it has reached epidemic proportions in Africa and is spreading rapidly in Asia. In contrast to the situation in Japan where, as referred to in another chapter, heterosexual transmission is very low (the same is true of the United States and Western Europe), in Africa and Asia it is very high. The reasons are not very clear, but probably have to do with the fact that most people who transmit the disease (prostitutes, in particular) are likely to have some other infectious disease also. Where this results in body sores that may be opened up during sexual intercourse, the virus would have access to the blood (as happens during anal intercourse between homosexuals, since the lining of the anus is rather fragile). As has been stressed earlier, HIV is pri-

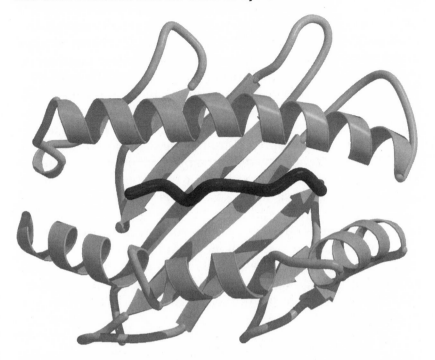

49. Display of virus molecules on cells. An 8 amino acid viral peptide derived from HIV (shown in dark) lying in the groove of part of an MHC protein (shown in grey) that is attached to the surface of a cell (not shown). The peptide is seen to lie on top of 4 diagonal, parallel strands of amino acids (called β sheet) and between 2 horizontal helical strands (called α helix) that form part of a human MHC molecule called HLA–B8. Regions of β sheet and α helix are typical of the way that chains of amino acids fold—largely as a result of hydrogen bonding—to form globular proteins. Photograph courtesy of Dr. C. A. O'Callaghan and Dr. Andrew McMichael of the Institute of Molecular Medicine, John Radcliffe Hospital, Oxford.

marily a blood-borne infection: The high incidence of HIV infection among intravenous drug users who share contaminated needles is proof of this. The second reason why a person infected with some other microbial disease is more likely to contract HIV in Africa (and elsewhere) is less well understood, but appears to be related to the general immune status of the individual: A primary infection that is not cured makes it easier for a second infection to take hold. Sometimes mistaken public measures exacerbate the situation. The politicians in the Indian state of Tamil Nadu, of which Madras (now called Chennai) is the capital, decided recently to bring all of the Tamil Nadu girls who were working the brothels of Bombay (now called Mumbai) back to their home state and to place them in other professions. The result? HIV infection, which had previously been virtually nonexistent in Tamil Nadu, spread through the state like wildfire.

Mention has been made of the problem of resistance to antibacterial drugs. Viruses, too, become resistant, in this case to the vaccines used against them. Resistant is perhaps not the right word, and insensitive would be better. For it is not so much a case of mutated viruses outgrowing others in the presence of some selective molecule like an antibiotic, but of viruses just mutating anyway. RNA viruses are especially liable to do this, since RNA synthesis is not checked by cellular control mechanisms as effectively as DNA synthesis. Influenza virus (an RNA virus) is a good example.

Influenza virus contains two proteins on its surface. One is required for binding to susceptible cells, the other is an enzyme that is required to release infective virus once it has replicated inside cells. The first protein is called hemagglutinin or H, because it agglutinates (clumps together) red cells (*haima* is Greek for "blood"). The second protein is called neuraminidase or N (attacking neuraminic acid). Neuraminic acid, a sugar residue that is present as part of a larger molecule on the surface membranes of our cells, is attacked by influenza virus; we shall return to this protein in Chapter 7 (Figure 61). Vaccines against influenza are directed mainly against the H protein. They are quite effective, but only for a number of years. Then a strain of virus having a slightly different structure of H will suddenly emerge, against which the original vaccine is no longer effective. The reasons for the emergence of new strains every so often are not clear. Suffice it to say that the influenza epidemics of 1918, 1957, and 1968 all had different H proteins on the surface of the virus. Viruses from the 1968 epidemic are still around. Interestingly there was also a mild epidemic in 1977, but this did not involve new strains: It infected only those born after 1957. In other words, those born before that date had acquired—and retained—sufficient immunity to fight off the infection. But to those who are not immune, influenza is a killer. More people died in their beds during the influenza epidemic of 1918 than the total number of men killed in the Great War that had just finished, even though the chances of an infantryman surviving on the battlefield were less than 1 in 10. Fortunately, knowledge of exactly what made the influenza virus of 1918 so virulent is at hand. A grave containing corpses of several people known to have died from influenza in 1918 has been identified in the Arctic region of northern Canada. Because the area is frozen most of the year, the corpses have decayed rather little. There is therefore a good chance that the particles of influenza virus that caused their deaths are still sufficiently intact to make it possible to determine the exact sequence of their genes, in other words their RNA, by modern technology. With permission from the relatives of the deceased, the corpses are now being exhumed. The information that analysis of the viral RNA will provide should help greatly in understanding the nature of virulence, and will lead to better design of influenza virus vaccines.

The immune system is extremely complex and our account so far has focused only on the bare essentials, as intricate as they may sound to anyone who is not a practicing immunologist! It must be mentioned that both B-cell-mediated secretion of immunoglobulins (against bacteria and other nonviral microbes) and T-cell-mediated destruction of virus-infected cells are stimulated by proteins called cytokines (giving energy to, i.e., stimulating, cells). Cytokines are like hormones; they are released by one type of cell to stimulate a second type of cell. Unlike the case of hormones, however, the sites of release and action are not distant organs, like pancreas and muscle in the case of insulin, or adrenals and liver in the case of epinephrine. The cells releasing cytokines and those responding to cytokines are present together—in the bloodstream, for example. Cytokines are released from T4 lymphocytes, also called helper cells. How are T4 cells stimulated in the first case? By a mechanism that is essentially the same as that involved in T cell killing of virus-infected cells. The cells involved in this instance are either B cells or macrophages (the phagocytic cells within tissues that are akin to the phagocytic cells in the circulation, namely, neutrophils). Any kind of foreign body—be it bacterium, protozoal parasite, or virus—that binds to B cells or macrophages is eventually internalized and degraded to small peptides. In the case of B cells this is in addition to the triggering of immunoglobulin release; in the case of macrophages it is part of the process that degrades the foreign molecules anyhow. The peptide binds to a groove in an MHC protein as described above and as illustrated in Figure 49. The MHC protein is not the same as the one that displays viral peptide to killer T cells (that is present on the surface of all cells); it is a close relative. The complex of peptide and MHC protein on the surface of B cells and macrophages is recognized by helper lymphocytes (T4 cells). The act of recognition causes the T4 cells to start secreting cytokines. It is T4 lymphocytes that are the primary target for HIV infection, which is why when these are knocked out, as in AIDS, both the B-cell system and the T-cell system suffer. As a result an AIDS patient cannot fight off *any* kind of microbial infection at all, whether bacterial, protozoal, or viral. Infections by fungi like *Candida* (fungi or yeasts are a "higher" form of bacterium that more closely resemble animal cells) are particularly serious as there are few drugs available to combat them. Normally *Candida* infections are not a problem, as they are kept down well by the immune system. Only when this is compromised, as in AIDS, do infections break out in places such as the mouth and the urinary tract. Such infections are known as thrush. Another consequence of AIDS is that patients have a higher than normal risk of developing cancer, particularly lymphomas (cancer of lymphocytes) and Kaposi's sarcoma, which are triggered by certain types of herpesvirus.

Why is this? Because several types of cancer cell are normally recognized and destroyed by the T-cell system that destroys virally infected cells. This depends, of course, on cancer cells producing "foreign" protein that is then degraded into peptides and presented on the surface of the cancer cell within the groove of an MHC protein like that depicted in Figure 49. But many cancer cells do not do this, which is why they evade such immune surveillance, as it is known. There is a viewpoint current among immunologists that immune surveillance of aberrant cells, like cancer cells, is a fundamental mechanism of all multi-celled organisms and that only later on in evolutionary time did it develop into the sophisticated system of defense against microbes. Ways of specifically boosting this part of the immune system is a particular goal of cancer therapy. The reader may wonder how the immune system distinguishes between "self" and "foreign" proteins. The mechanism is not clear, but we know that it occurs when the immune system is being laid down, in late pregnancy and infancy. This is why infants, whose immune system has not yet formed, are particularly at risk of infection, though they acquire some resistance through the ingestion of immunoglobulins in their mother's milk; this is a very good reason for breast feeding. Any protein that escapes detection at this crucial time in infancy will subsequently be considered as foreign by the immune system. If it appears in the circulation it will set up a B-cell response. In other words B lymphocytes bearing an immunoglobulin molecule complementary to the protein will bind it and eventually destroy it, and any cell on which it is displayed will be attacked. Equally, cells displaying a peptide derived from such a protein that is recognized as "foreign" will set up a T-cell response. These cells, too, will be attacked and destroyed. Such mechanisms may contribute to autoimmune diseases, to be described shortly.

One of the first cytokines to be discovered was the protein interferon. Recall that cytokines are hormonelike proteins that are secreted by one type of cell and that act on another type of cell. The name interferon was coined to denote interference with a viral infection, after it was noted that when a cell becomes infected with a virus, it secretes a particular protein. Interferon protects further cells from being infected by the virus. At least this is what happens to isolated cells studied in the laboratory. As is so often the case, extrapolation to the human body tells another story. Interferon has been tested as an antiviral therapy on people with a variety of different viral infections. The results have been consistently disappointing. Partly this is because high doses of interferon are quite toxic. Interferon was initially found to prevent the synthesis of viral proteins in infected cells, which is presumably how it works. But it is now known to inhibit the synthesis of *all* proteins in the infected cell; in other words to inhibit "good," i.e., host proteins, as well as "bad," i.e., viral proteins. This makes it a potentially toxic molecule. However, this is not the end of the story. Because of its inhibitory properties, interferon has been tested against various types of cancer: Surprisingly, after all, some beneficial effects have been reported. The exact opposite happened with idoxuridine, a molecule that was initially synthesized as a potential inhibitor of DNA synthesis in cancer cells. This is because it is an analogue of thymine (T), one of the nucleotide building blocks of DNA (the molecular differences between analogues and building blocks are illustrated in Figure 60 in Chapter 7). Idoxuridine proved pretty ineffective against cancer cells. Nonetheless, by chance someone tried it on herpesvirus-infected cells (herpes being a DNA virus). It proved remarkably effective and is now in routine use to treat herpes infections of the cornea. Phosphoamides (to which we shall return in Chapter 7) were developed as war gases, but were found by chance to be effective against certain leukemias. There is a valuable lesson here for those who fund medical research: Do not be too restrictive in supporting only projects that have a chance of success based on current expectations. The unexpected result often leads to a breakthrough in an entirely different area. There is indeed a place for "blue skies" research.

A question that has already been raised in a previous chapter concerns the variation from person to person in their response to different diseases. In the case of microbial infections, we are beginning to understand one reason. It will be recalled that MHC proteins fall not just into two main classes, those on all cells of the body (except red blood cells) and those restricted to B lymphocytes and macrophages, but that within each class there is much person-to-person variation, which accounts for transplant rejection between all individuals other than identical twins. MHC proteins are, in fact, the most varied molecules in our body, more so even than the 100 million different immunoglobulins capable of being made by any one person. A few years ago a team of scientists from Oxford University went into The Gambia in tropical west Africa to find out why some people seem to be resistant to malaria, whereas others come down with the disease. A previous study, many years earlier, had shown that individuals who carry the sickle cell gene (responsible for making an aberrant hemoglobin) are at an advantage over those who have normal hemoglobin, because the malarial parasite is less able to survive in red blood cells that contain sickle-cell hemoglobin, than in normal red blood cells. In the case of the Gambians, all of the individuals tested had normal hemoglobin, so this possibility for varying susceptibility to malaria was eliminated. What the team found was that some of those who were able to resist the ravages of the disease—even though they were obviously bitten by *Plasmodium falciparum*-infected mosquitoes as much as other groups—have a particular type of MHC protein (HLA-B53) on the surface of their cells. When the scientists investigated what peptides—containing 8–10 amino acids—fit into the groove of this protein, they found that only 9 peptides out of some 60 tested, do so. Next they measured the ability of cytotoxic (killer) T cells, isolated from the Gambian volunteers, to destroy cells to which one of those 9 peptides had been added. The result? Cell killing occurred only with just one of the 9 peptides tested. That particular peptide forms part of a *P. falciparum* protein that is made by the parasite when it is inside the liver of an infected person (the parasite divides in the liver before it infects the red blood cells). What this research shows is how person-to-person variation—a subtle difference in the proteins that constitute the MHC system—can account for person-to-person variation in resistance to infectious disease. An added bonus of the work is that it has pointed to a candidate molecule, the protein that contains the active peptide, from which to construct a vaccine.

We have already seen that infants are very prone to microbial infections because their immune system is not yet fully developed. But why are the old also more susceptible? Why is influenza sometimes known as "the old man's way to the grave" and why is influenza vaccination recommended for the over-60s? It is because the human body, like any other machine, tends to wear out with time and its ability to carry out the many complicated reactions that constitute the immune response gradually declines. The severely malnourished are less able to mount a successful immune response at any age. There is in addition a very specific reason why our immune system declines with age, and it concerns the T cells. Like all of the white (and red) blood cells, T lymphocytes are made in the bone marrow. In order to mature and build up the tremendous repertoire of cells able to recognize one out of 100 million different molecules, T cells are processed by the thymus, a small organ in the upper part of the chest. The thymus, however, begins to decline already in childhood, and by early adulthood is virtually nonexistent. After this time, any failure of the system is irreparable.

There are several situations when we may wish to dampen down our immune system. The rejection of organ transplants is one. Two other situations concern allergy and autoimmune disease. Most of us are allergic to some substances that are breathed in, eaten, or that enter by way of the skin (Table 5). Typical of the first category is pollen, which is a major cause of asthma afflicting 150 million people worldwide; hay fever, rhinitis (runny nose), and more severe symptoms are other consequences. House dust and cat fur are other common causes. The second category includes gluten (a constituent of flour and bakery products), shell-

Table 5. Some Common Allergens

Through nose
Pollen
Car fumes
House dust (including mites)
Cat fur
Feathers
Through mouth
Gluten
Shellfish
Peanut oil
Chocolate
Drugs (antibiotics; β-blockers)
Through skin
Poison ivy
Nettles
Bee stings (and other insects)

A list of all known allergens would be virtually endless.

fish, some antibiotics like penicillin, and a host of other compounds that cause vomiting and other symptoms. The third category includes poison ivy and nettles, some washing powders, as well as the sting of bees and other insects, all of which result in skin rashes or wheals, and can also lead to eczema.

The reason for most allergic responses is the presence of a particular class of immunoglobulins on the surface of mast cells, which are found in most tissues, which is why the consequences can involve the respiratory tract, the gut, or the skin. It should be mentioned that immunoglobulins fall into different classes—called isotypes—depending on their exact structure. All immunoglobulins are made up of light and heavy chains, and each of these chains consists of variable and constant regions, exactly as described earlier. The features by which one class or isotype differs from another are in the composition of the constant region in its heavy chains. The immunoglobulin on the surface of mast cells is called immunoglobulin E, in contrast to the immunoglobulin on B cells, which is called M. The immunoglobulin that is released into the circulation following stimulation of a B cell is called G. There is another class of immunoglobulin, called A, in mucus secretions and mother's milk. Immunoglobulin A, like immunoglobulins M and G, is concerned with conferring immunity; immunoglobulin E is part of the allergic response. In that instance, the irritant molecule, appropriately called an allergen, reacts with immunoglobulin E in precisely the same way that a molecule or foreign particle binds to an immunoglobulin M molecule on the surface of a B lymphocyte. Again, the analogy is with a key—the allergen—fitting into just one of hundreds, actually 100 million, of different locks—the immunoglobulin E on the mast cell. In short, just as the variety of different immunoglobulin-bearing B lymphocytes is enormous, so the number of different immunoglobulins on mast cells is also enormous, enabling widely different allergens to be recognized. What is different, of course, is the consequence of recognition: In the case of B lymphocytes, the consequence is beneficial since it leads to the elimination of the invading molecule, whereas in the case of mast cells the consequence is detrimental since it leads to an allergic response (Figure 50). The allergic reaction that is initiated within

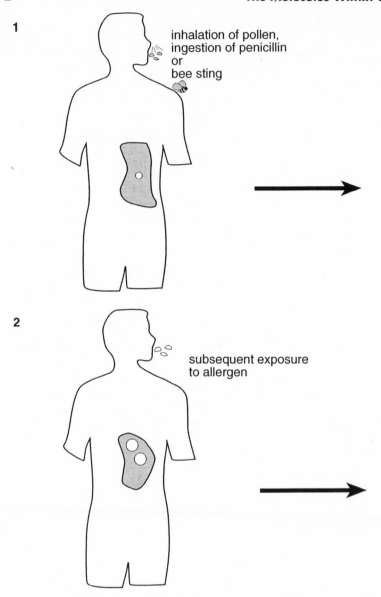

50. The immune response in allergy. Note the similarity between the response to allergens—which leads to hypersensitivity, i.e., to our detriment—and the response to infectious agents (Figure 48)—which leads to protection, i.e., to our benefit. From *An Introduction to Human Biochemistry* by C. A. Pasternak, Oxford University Press, 1979.

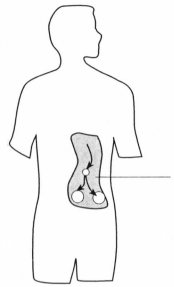

stimulation of lymphocytes

slight allergic reaction

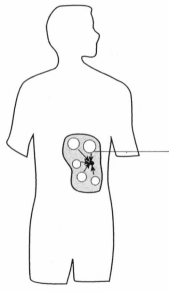

histamine release: skin rash;
anaphylactic shock; etc.

severe allergic reaction

50. (*continued*)

the mast cell culminates in the release of a number of different molecules, chief of which is histamine. It is for this reason that antihistamine drugs are effective in many situations. Histamine is a compound that acts both as a hormone and as a neurotransmitter (its molecular structure is shown in Figure 73 in Chapter 8). When the reaction is in the respiratory tract, histamine causes constriction of the airways (which makes breathing difficult), running nose, sneezing, and so forth. In the gut it causes vomiting and in the skin, the local reaction of rashes and wheals. But the consequences can be much more severe: bowel disease, anaphylactic shock (the body's reaction to certain foreign molecules) leading to heart failure and even death. This is because some 10% of the population—the figure has been put as high as 25%—has exceptionally high amounts of immunoglobulin E. The cause is the function of certain inherited genes that control the amount of immunoglobulin E that is made. The result in such people is that even the tiniest amount of allergen can initiate a reaction. That reaction, in hypersensitive individuals, is not only severe, it is also very broad: An allergen that enters the body through the gut will affect the skin and respiratory tracts as well, causing rhinitis, asthma, and eczema in addition to vomiting and bowel symptoms; an allergen that is breathed in or enters via the skin will likewise affect all other organs. Moreover, someone who is hypersensitive to one allergen is likely to be hypersensitive to many others as well: to penicillin as well as to bee stings, to cat mites as well as to shellfish, and so forth. The list is endless (Table 5) and contains quite unexpected molecules. The oil from peanuts (the rogue molecule, probably a protein, has not yet been identified) can constitute so strong an allergen that a hypersensitive baby can react to breast feeding if its mother has eaten a peanut butter sandwich. Moreover a boy had to be hospitalized for 2 days after someone on an airplane, sitting two rows behind him, had eaten peanuts with his cocktail (the boy's mother, aware of her son's hypersensitivity, had asked the stewardess not to serve nuts to any of the passengers sitting near them, but it is difficult to persuade the average airline staff to deny an entire 747 jumbo jet a snack with their cocktails because of a single passenger). Merely inhaling trace amounts of vapor from the nuts triggered a full-scale allergic reaction.

The list of potential allergens—from chocolate and avocado to latex and feathers—and the number of sufferers appears to be increasing. Why should this be? The atmosphere in our cities is becoming more polluted, house dust mites, one of the most common causes, may be on the increase as more people keep cats and dogs as pets inside their houses, and we spend more time indoors or in cars instead of in the fresh air of the countryside. All of these may be contributory factors, but the truth is that we really do not know the answer; at least, though, we are becoming aware of the problem.

Or are we? Every so often, one still hears of someone who is allergic to bee stings and, when stung, rapidly takes himself off to the casualty department of the nearest hospital. Unless on the ball, the normal reaction of the admitting nurse is "sit down and wait"; by the time the physician arrives, the patient is dead. People who know that they are hypersensitive should always carry a small first-aid kit in their pocket or purse, since bee stings generally happen far away from hospitals anyway. The kit contains a syringe already filled with epinephrine (called adrenaline outside the United States) which should be injected immediately into the soft tissue of one's buttock, and a tablet of antihistamine, which should be taken at the same time. The treatment is effective for other allergies also, because the precipitating cause—a massive release of histamine—is the same. One does not become acclimatized to these allergic reactions; on the contrary, they get worse at each exposure as the body becomes ever more sensitive. What to do? Alternative medicine has entered the arena: In Hyderabad, India, asthmatics are lining up to have a small (2 inches long) live fish known as a murrel that has had its mouth filled with special herbs, dropped down their throats. As the fish wriggles downwards it obligingly dislodges phlegm in the esophagus; on arrival in the stomach beneficial herbs are released (and the fish dies). The power of belief in alternative medicine is very strong: The fact that asthma is caused by an accumulation of phlegm in the lungs (in narrow tubes called bronchioles, to be precise), not in the esophagus, seems not to matter. If the treatment is causing you to shiver with distaste, be heartened: One fish per year, for 3 successive years, is said to provide a lifelong cure. For most of us, though, antihistamine tablets, bronchodilatory preparations containing steroids, and—most effective of all—avoidance of known allergens wherever possible, remains the best treatment currently available. For asthmatics, a novel treatment that involves no drugs may be at hand. A device through which one breathes, strengthens the muscles involved with continued use—a sort of physiotherapy for breathing—and has been found effective in elderly people who suffer from shortness of breath. Researchers at Birmingham University in England have now found that the device provides relief for sufferers from asthma also. An alternate solution is to desensitize oneself against the allergen to which one is, or has become, sensitive. This is not as straightforward as it sounds. First, each allergen is a different molecule and since each immunoglobulin E—like other immunoglobulins—reacts against just one particular molecule, the desensitization process has to be repeated over and over for every rogue allergen. Second, each desensitization is a lengthy procedure because only minute amounts of allergen can be given at any one time; recall the problem of *increased* sensitivity after each exposure mentioned above. The ideal solution, of course, is to suppress the synthesis of immunoglobulin E in our body. So far, such specific immunosuppression has not been achieved.

Autoimmunity is also caused by an excessive immune response. In this instance, as in graft rejection, it is B and T lymphocytes that are the problem. These classes of white cells in our body are also, as we saw earlier on, involved in the immune response against infectious microbes. In short, our immune system is balanced on a knife edge: Too little response, and we fall prey to the first influenza virus, *Streptococcus* bacterium, malarial parasite, or *Candida* fungus that attacks us; too much response, and we develop an autoimmune disease. For reasons that are not yet clear, the lymphocytes mount an attack not against a foreign molecule, but against one of the body's own proteins. Normally any lymphocyte that is directed against such a protein is eliminated by the thymus very early on in life. But sometimes a protein is missed, or a protein that is not normally exposed becomes exposed for one reason or another. Currently the most likely explanation, however, is that one of our proteins becomes recognized as foreign because it happens to resemble the protein of an infecting microbe against which an immune response has been mounted. Cells that display such proteins are then attacked by T lymphocytes and by circulating immunoglobulins. This is the underlying cause of damage to specific tissues like thyroid, adrenals, stomach, pancreas, muscle, and others (Table 6). As with allergies, there is a strong genetic element, which can account for up to 50% of cases. Some examples of autoimmune diseases and the types of molecule that are involved follow.

The thyroid, a small organ at the base of our neck, provides a good illustration for two reasons: first, because it was one of the earliest organs to be associated with autoimmune disease, and we now know a great deal about thyroid problems in molecular terms; second, because the thyroid provides a good example of how hormones work. One effect of an autoimmune attack on the thyroid is to prevent the organ from releasing thyroid hormones. These are two amino-acid-like molecules that are derived by breakdown of thyroglobulin, an iodine-containing protein that is made within the cells of the thyroid. One of the amino-acid-like molecules contains three atoms of iodine and is known as T3; the

Table 6. Autoimmune Diseases

Recognition of molecules in specific cells	
Affected organ or tissue	Outcome
Thyroid	Myxedema
	Thyrotoxicosis
Pancreas	Diabetes
Adrenal	Addison's disease
Stomach	Pernicious anemia
Muscle	Myasthenia gravis
Brain	Multiple sclerosis
Red cells	Hemolytic anemia
Recognition of molecules in circulation	
Immune complexes	Rheumatoid arthritis
DNA	SLE (systemic lupus erythematosus)

Recognition of certain molecules in specific cells leads to the stimulation of an organ or tissue, as in thyrotoxicosis, or to the destruction of an organ or tissue, as in all other cases.

other contains four atoms of iodine and is known as T4 or thyroxine. Together these two hormones control many physiological processes, of which the most important is metabolic rate: Too much T3 and/or T4 in our blood, and we burn up nutrients fast and become hyperactive. If not treated, thyrotoxicosis (Graves' disease) develops, characterized by a rapid heartbeat, sweating, intolerance to heat, increased appetite yet loss of weight; the eyes often appear quite prominent. Too little, and metabolic rate decreases: We become sluggish and lethargic. If not treated, myxedema (also known as Hashimoto's disease or thyroiditis) develops, in which the skin becomes dry and coarse, the patient tends to gain weight and to show an intolerance to cold; mental activity is dulled. Autoimmunity is only one cause of myxedema, or for that matter of the other diseases to be described. In the case of myxedema, for example, lack of iodine in the diet is another cause. The English crime writer Dorothy Sayers wrote a story about a villain who deliberately keeps his victim, who has myxedema, deprived of thyroxine (T4). She becomes sluggish, her skin hardens, and she becomes quite like a tired animal slouching around the house. Then the villain will add some thyroxine tablets to her food so that she temporarily recovers and becomes another person (shades of Jekyll and Hyde, though in that case not related to thyroid insufficiency). The point of the story is to show that one can often reverse changes in thyroid function relatively easily: in cases of iodine deficiency by giving iodine, more often by augmenting or inhibiting T3 and T4 in the bloodstream. In the case of myxedema, the molecule that is recognized during an autoimmune attack on the thyroid is the iodinated protein thyroglobulin, from which T3 and T4 are released. Destruction of thyroglobulin, then, leads to myxedema. But the opposite effect—an increased production of T3 and T4, leading to thyrotoxicosis—can also occur. In this instance the immune target is a protein on the surface of thyroid cells that is the receptor for another hormone. That hormone is a protein called thyroid stimulating hormone or TSH. TSH is secreted from the pituitary gland (in the brain) in response to circulating T3 and T4: if levels of T3 and T4 fall, more TSH is produced. If levels of T3 and T4 rise, less TSH is produced. The way that TSH controls the release of T3 and T4 from the thyroid is as follows. TSH binds to a receptor on thyroid cells: Much TSH, and the thyroid cells are stimulated into releasing much T3 and T4; little TSH, and the release of T3 and T4 from the thyroid is depressed. In this way the levels of T3 and T4 are normally kept within strict limits. This type of control mechanism—called feedback or homeostasis—is typical of all hormone action. In the case of autoimmune thyrotoxicosis, an immunoglobulin molecule comes to recognize the TSH receptor on thyroid cells and binds to it, as though it were TSH. The result? The thyroid is fooled into thinking that there is TSH bound on its surface, and therefore responds by releasing more T3 and T4. Left uncontrolled, thyrotoxicosis ensues. Thus does molecular mimicry lead to disease.

Another example of an autoimmune disorder involving hormones is diabetes. In this instance the hormone is insulin, a relatively small protein (its small size made it the first protein to have its structure, that is, the sequence of its amino acids, determined). The molecule that "senses" whether more or less insulin is to be released is glucose. A high level of glucose, like after a meal, stimulates insulin release from the pancreas. The insulin that is released acts to lower blood glucose, by stimulating utilization of glucose by liver, heart, muscle, and adipose tissue. As glucose levels fall, secretion of insulin from the pancreas is depressed. In type I diabetes, the cells of the pancreas that produce insulin are destroyed, and insulin cannot be released in response to a high glucose level. Unlike the situation just described for thyroid deficiency or excess, the molecular nature of the immune attack is not at all clear. Indeed, the reason for regarding diabetes as an autoimmune disease is still largely circumstantial. It is to be noted that in type II diabetes, which can be controlled without having to provide extra insulin by injection, the release of insulin from the pancreas is only slightly impaired; the main cause of the problem is resistance to the insulin that *is* released into the bloodstream.

Several other diseases are, or may be, the result of an autoimmune attack on certain tissues and organs. In Addison's disease, in which the patient suffers from weakness, loss of energy, and low blood pressure, the function of the adrenal cortex is impaired. This is a small organ (see Figure 20 in Chapter 3) that produces steroid hormones (recall that steroids are molecules made from cholesterol). These hormones—cortisol is one—control body processes like inflammation, water excretion in the kidney, carbohydrate metabolism, and others. Immune attack against a protein called intrinsic factor that resides on the surface of certain cells that line the stomach and that help to absorb vitamin B_{12}, leads to pernicious anemia. This disease is characterized by a decreased production of red blood cells, caused by lack of vitamin B_{12}. Immune attack against a receptor protein for acetylcholine—a neurotransmitter (see Chapter 8) that is situated on the surface of muscle cells—leads to myasthenia gravis. This disease is characterized by dysfunction of the eyelids (initially), followed by the failure of muscle in arms, legs, and throat. If not treated, patients die of asphyxia. This is because breathing stops, the result of the unresponsiveness (to acetylcholine) of the chest muscles. Another autoimmune disease that involves the failure of neurotransmitter molecules to activate their targets is multiple sclerosis. In this case there is a progressive failure of muscle and other organs to respond to neuronal signals. Attack against a molecule on the surface of red cells leads to hemolytic anemia, characterized by loss of red blood cells (similar in outcome, if not in cause, to pernicious anemia).

The autoimmune situations we have mentioned so far are all examples of attack against a specific tissue or group of cells. In most cases, the ensuing diseases can be treated according to the molecular defect: in the case of myxedema, by giving T3 and T4; in the case of thyrotoxicosis, by giving anti-T3/T4 drugs; in the case of Addison's disease, by giving steroids; in the case of pernicious anemia, by giving additional B_{12}; in the case of diabetes, by giving insulin; in the case of myasthenia gravis, by giving drugs that inhibit the enzyme that degrades acetylcholine (hence potentiating the action of acetylcholine); in the case of hemolytic anemia, by giving blood transfusions; no satisfactory treatment is currently available for multiple sclerosis. Some of the symptoms of AIDS (despite the name of acquired immune *deficiency* syndrome) are suggestive of an autoimmune reaction; again no satisfactory treatment is currently available.

Two types of autoimmune disease, which are quite common, are directed not against any one tissue, but lead to disseminated tissue damage. The first is characterized by immunoglobulins recognizing and binding to other immunoglobulins. In this case the variable part of one molecule binds to the constant part of another, in piggyback fashion. Such an immunoglobulin–immunoglobulin complex encourages the binding of a third molecule. This is one of the proteins of the complement cascade, which was mentioned earlier in relation to the killing of bacteria by forming a leaky plug in their membrane. Such complexes of immunoglobulin and complement protein are called immune complexes. They circulate freely in the bloodstream, but tend to deposit in joints and elsewhere, leading to inflammation and rheumatoid arthritis. The second situation is similar, and even more widespread. In this instance it is DNA that somehow becomes recognized by immunoglobulins that forms immune complexes. These lead to inflammation and damage to many different organs: Muscles and joints are the most common tissues affected in this disease, termed systemic lupus erythematosus (SLE or lupus). Other affected sites in lupus are the heart and respiratory system, the kidney (glomerulonephritis is the most common cause of death in SLE), the nervous system, and so forth. As with rheumatoid arthritis, there is no specific treatment that can be targeted against the molecular defect, and sufferers have to resort to treatment by anti-inflammatory drugs such as steroids.

———————◆———————

This chapter has described the body's defense to microbial infections. It has stressed the fact that we are able to mount a specific response to virtually any molecule we are likely to meet. Whether an invading microbe is able to initiate a serious infection or is eliminated before it can do so, depends on a delicate balance between the virulence of the microbe and the effectiveness of our immune system. There is another balance: between destruction by the immune system of foreign invaders, and destruction of our own cells, leading to autoimmune disease. We spend our lives walking on a knife edge, poised between health and disease: Fortunately for us the knife tilts somewhat in favor of health, at least for the first three score and ten years of our lives.

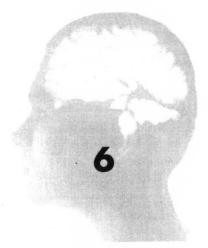

6

STRESS

THE MIND–BODY RELATIONSHIP

———————◆———————

Stress is *the* illness of our age. It is on the lips of psychiatrists, sociologists, and physicians, of clerics, homeopaths, and executives. Everything from health foods and vacations to furniture and cosmetics is advertised as "reducing stress." What is stress, and how can we treat it? We may define stress along the lines proposed by Hans Selye. An innovative Hungarian scientist living in Canada, Selye considered stress to be any condition in which there is an imbalance between environmental demands and our body's capability—including, of course, our mind—to meet them. Such situations, Selye proposed, ultimately lead to disease. Few would argue with him today, though 20 years ago these were rather novel ideas. Where our body *is* capable of meeting demands, sometimes referred to as *mild* stress—like rigorous exercise, appearing on television, or clinching a business deal—the effects can be beneficial, not deleterious. This state of affairs may be compared with the immune system: A response sufficient to destroy an invading microbe is beneficial; an excessive response, leading to autoimmune disease, is detrimental.

Everyone has experienced stress: at work, at home, at school, at play; the pressure to succeed, the disappointment of failure, the breakup of a relationship, the death of a loved one, the difficulty of making ends meet, the loss of a job. If asked to gauge the degree of stress in each of these circumstances, one comes up— on average—with a list such as that of Table 7. As attitudes of society change, so the degree of certain stresses changes also: being a homosexual at the end of the twentieth century is less stressful than it was in 1950, but being unable to afford an automobile is probably more stressful today than it was 50 years ago. If asked to say what part of our body experiences stress, the answer would undoubtedly be the mind, and this is clearly where the stresses discussed so far originate. And while most people would agree that stress is somehow debilitating, and that particular stresses such as pressure at work can result in a peptic ulcer, they would be surprised to learn that stress can lead to a whole variety of diseases, including diabetes, heart attack, and even cancer. Yet this is precisely the case, as reported by various clinicians in the following paragraphs.

"Bereavement has often been cited as a factor contributing to the initiation of cancer, tuberculosis, diabetes, lymphomas and leukemias, and heart failure" (Weiner, 1987). "Intense or unusual emotional stress, often involving anger, is associated with arrhythmia onset (abnormality of heartbeat) in approximately 20% of cases. These observations shed light on the possible role of psychological factors in the pathogenesis of sudden cardiac death" (Reich, 1985). A warning to pregnant mothers not merely to give up cigarettes—assuming they have not already done so— excessive alcohol, and many types of pills, but also to try to come to terms with their in-laws: "Guilt, anxiety and stress are detrimental to mental health and can cause neuroendocrine changes [i.e., involving neurotransmitters and hormones] harmful to fetal development" (Rossett and Weiner, 1985). These quotations illustrate the kind of diseases that have been associated with stress. The disease for which an association with stress is strongest is undoubtedly heart disease. A particularly convincing study was a recent one carried out in Germany on "blue-collar" workers. It is becoming generally clear that those lower down the ladder suf-

Table 7. Degrees of Stress

Event	Finnish LCU weight
Health	
Recent illness (in bed for a week or hospitalization)	62
Change in heavy physical work or exercise	19
Change in sleeping habits	15
Change in eating habits	11
Work	
Recently out of work	50
Recently fired from work	50
Retirement from farming, forestry, or industry	40
Change to new type of work	36
Change in work responsibilities	29
Troubles with boss	22
Work or life going well (e.g., awards, achievements)	20
Correspondence course (home study)	17
Change in hours of work a day	13
Home and family	
Concern over health of family member	54
Recently married	50
Separation from wife because of marital problems	48
Gaining a new family member (in the home)	39
Separation from wife because of work	34
Engaged to be married	32
New home improvements	26
Son or daughter leaving home	23
Wife began or ended work	23
Troubles with in-laws	22
Change in get-togethers with friends	21
Change to a new residence	15
Change in get-togethers with relatives	13
Vacation	11
Personal and Social	
Death of wife	105
Divorce	80
Held in jail	64
Sexual difficulties	41
Change in number of arguments with wife	40
Death of a close relative	39
Financial difficulties	38
Major decisions regarding the future	38
Death of a close friend	34
Unpaid bills leading to threatened legal action	26
Recent purchases worth more than 8000 FMk ($2000)	22
Change in religious or political convictions	20
Change in personal habits	12
Recent purchases worth less than 8000 FMk	11
Minor violations of the law	7

One hundred fifty healthy Finnish men and women were asked to assess the degree of stress brought about by various changes in their lifestyle. The results were pooled and are expressed as arbitrary Life-Change Unit (LCU) weights. Adapted from a paper by R. H. Rahe, L. Bennett, M. Romo, P. Siltanen, and R. J. Arthur in *American Journal of Psychiatry*, **130**, 1222, 1973.

fer more from occupational stress than those higher up: Their job satisfaction is lower, they suffer more from financial worries, their fear of unemployment is greater. As mentioned earlier, the stress of making high-flying deals is often more beneficial than harmful. The German study, carried out by Johannes Siegrist, showed that middle-aged men suffering from occupational stress had a threefold higher incidence of heart attacks than those without the symptoms of stress. Similar results are being found in China. Not only does stress lead to disease, it may worsen the course of those already ill. The Los Angeles earthquake in January 1994, which was one of the strongest earthquakes ever to hit a major city in North America, provides a good example of the effects of this kind of stress. The rate of sudden deaths from a heart attack in patients with atherosclerosis jumped more than fivefold on the day of the earthquake. Over the following 6 days, the rate returned to what it had been before the earthquake. The conclusion that the emotional stress of the earthquake precipitated cardiac death in some who might otherwise have lived is inescapable.

The earliest, and most common, consequences of stress are insomnia on the one hand, and mild aches and pains in the back, shoulder, neck, and lower limbs on the other. They are obviously linked, since muscle pain or fibrositis is often strong enough to prevent normal sleep. The opposite is also true: Impaired sleep can lead to fibrositis.

There is another aspect of stress, which is that it can originate outside the mind as well as within it. We now know that an infectious disease, a surgical operation, even intense exercise, can lead to the same changes as psychological stress. Of course it has long been suspected that if one is run-down or depressed, one is more liable to catch a cold or other infection, but proof was lacking. This was supplied by a study at the Common Cold Unit near Salisbury in England (now closed down, but for financial reasons, not for lack of scientific rectitude). Volunteers were inoculated with the common cold virus or with influenza virus and their symptoms—runny nose, excretion of more virus, and so forth—monitored. At the same time their lifestyle over the previous 6 months was assessed. It was found that those who had experienced a stressful event like bereavement, divorce, or loss of job developed worse colds than those who had not; even mild anxiety or depression correlated with a more intense cold.

Another type of stress accompanies a surgical operation. Following surgery, the body is in a state of shock that is similar to that following a car crash or falling off a ladder. Normally the shock—a classical stress stimulus—is treated merely with sedatives and the patient recovers. But if it is not, the tissues of the body may remain affected through various hormonal imbalances and this constitutes a risk factor for further disease. In addition, having to stay in a hospital is a recognized stress factor that may be compounded by emotional and hormonal stresses in operations such as a hysterectomy.

Exercise is not generally regarded as stressful. On the contrary, moderate exercise is undoubtedly beneficial to mind as well as to body. Already 2000 years ago the Romans recognized this: *Mens sana in corpore sano* ("A healthy mind in a healthy body"). But whereas moderate exercise is entirely beneficial, excessive exercise has the opposite effect. Of course it is not surprising that professional athletes are as prone to emotional stress as anyone else leading a highly competitive lifestyle. But what is now becoming clear is that physical overexertion itself is a cause of stress and that the consequence is often an increased susceptibility to infection. An example concerns the British former Olympic long-distance runner Sebastian Coe. It was a respiratory infection—as well as repeated bouts of toxoplasmosis (a protozoal disease caused by eating uncooked meat and from contact with domestic pets like cats)—brought on by bouts of hard training, that led to his failing to even qualify for the Seoul Olympics in 1988. The link between the stress of muscular activity and infection involves a depressed immune system: Measurement of white cells and molecules such as immunoglobulins, cytokines, and so forth in elite athletes during training shows that some striking changes (Table 8) result from slight damage to heavily exercised muscle. They revert to normal within 24 hours following rest. Such changes do not occur following moderate training or exercise. While immune

Table 8. Immune Consequences of Heavy Exercise

Infiltration of phagocytes (neutrophils and macrophages) to sites of muscular activity

Activation of phagocytes: free radical formation

Release of certain cytokines at sites of muscular activity

Decrease of immunoglobulins in blood, saliva, and nasal washings

Suppression of killer and other lymphocytes

Some of the changes of immune function that have been recorded following a stressful bout of physical activity are listed. Adapted from *Physical Activity, Training and the Immune Response* by R. J. Shephard, Cooper Publishing Group, 1997.

function is low, the athlete is at risk of an infection. Several of the changes in immune function can be detected by analysis of saliva, sampling that causes no discomfort to the athlete. By careful monitoring, training sessions can be phased so as to ensure that immune function has returned to normal before the next session is started.

Just as stress increases susceptibility to infectious disease, so an infection is itself a type of stress stimulus. This has so far been studied mainly at the level of isolated cells, but appears to apply as well to the body as a whole. If cells are exposed to a stressful environment, such as abnormal heat or cold, an infecting virus, or the presence of noxious chemicals, they respond in a number of characteristic ways. One way is to synthesize a group of proteins called heat shock or stress proteins. One of their functions is to enable stressed cells to recover and to become protected against a second insult. Another response is to increase the uptake of glucose into cells; again this may help to fight off the effects of environmental stress. Both responses are beneficial, so here we have an example of molecular changes that are compatible with the observation that mild forms of stress—a little excitement, some mental stimulation, a certain degree of physical exercise—are beneficial and lead to a prolonged and healthy life.

The most common molecular change brought about by stress is an increased secretion of two hormones: epinephrine (adrenaline) and cortisol (hydrocortisone). Both are synthesized and stored in the adrenal gland (see Figure 20 on p. 56): epinephrine in the part called the medulla, and cortisol in the part called the cortex. Epinephrine secretion is triggered by nerve impulses coming from the brain; cortisol secretion is also triggered in the brain, but in this instance the message is transmitted not through nerves but through a hormone—adrenocorticotropic hormone or ACTH—that is secreted from the brain (ACTH secretion is itself stimulated by epinephrine). Such mind–body cross talk is illustrated in Figure 51. It has been known for half a century that epinephrine is released when someone becomes frightened and that it stimulates the breakdown of glycogen from muscle and liver, so as to make available the extra energy required for the sudden muscular movement of running away. Epinephrine has therefore been regarded as the "fear and flight" or "fear and fight" hormone. Nervous apprehension like an impending examination or public speech, anxiety about missing a train or air flight, receipt of a letter from a bank manager or the Inland Revenue Service (tax inspector in Europe), being arrested in a police state, certainly provoke fear, but where is the flight? Running to catch a train or to avoid arrest may involve extra muscular activity, but opening a letter does not. The need for energy for flight is probably something we have inherited from our ancestors: It is pretty important for a gazelle to start running at top speed the moment it espies a lion. For its part, the lion probably has an epinephrine surge, too. What we do know is that epinephrine also causes an increase in heartbeat, sweating, and bowel movement—the well-known "butterflies" of nervous apprehension. An occasional increase causes no lasting damage; it is when one's whole lifestyle is dominated by fear and apprehension that ulcers and other ailments develop: currency traders beware!

A quantitative assessment of "butterflies" has been achieved by the following experiment. Volunteers had earphones placed over their ears. The earphones were attached to a machine that transmitted pieces of poetry and other forms of literature. The machine transmitted the same piece into each ear, or it transmitted a different piece into each ear. The subjects were then asked to write down—as best they could—what they had heard. At the same time the movement of fluid in their gut was measured by

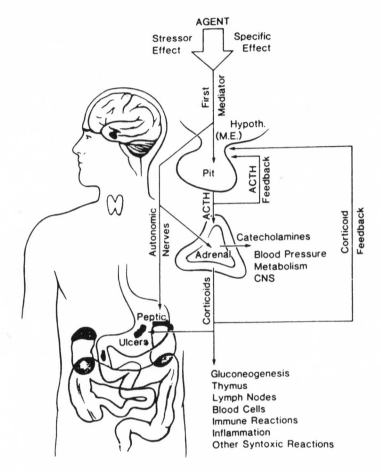

51. Mind–body cross talk. Electrical impulses from the hypothalamus in the brain reach the pituitary (also in the brain). Here they are translated into chemical signals, like the protein hormone ACTH, that act on the adrenal. This releases further hormones to various parts of the body: catecholamines (epinephrine and norepinephrine) and corticoids like cortisol. From *The Stress Concept: Past, Present and Future* by Hans Selye, McGraw–Hill, 1977.

routine surgical techniques. The results were clear-cut: When the same piece was transmitted into each ear and the subjects had no difficulty in recalling it, fluid movement was normal; when the transmission into each ear was different and the subjects became confused and had difficulty in recalling each piece, fluid movement was altered, compatible with mild diarrhea (Figure 52).

The relationship of cortisol secretion and stress is illustrated by the following experiment. As mentioned in a previous chapter, one of the actions of cortisol—like that of epinephrine—is to in-

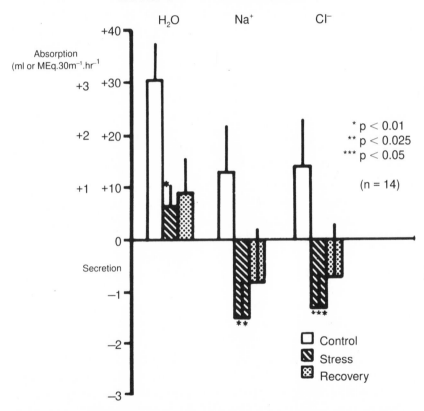

EFFECT OF DICHOTOMOUS LISTENING STRESS ON NET TRANSPORT IN HUMAN JEJUNUM

52. Stress and the intestine. Volunteers with earphones were subjected to stress as described in the text. Prior to the stress (control), during the stress (stress), and immediately afterwards (recovery), the absorption from, or secretion into, the small intestine (jejunum) of water (H_2O), sodium (Na^+), and chloride (Cl^-) was measured. The results are the averages of 14 separate experiments. Data kindly supplied by Dr. L. A. Turnberg.

crease energy supply; in this instance by stimulating the release of fatty acids from adipose cells by triglyceride breakdown. The experiment went as follows. Parachute trainees were asked to assess their degree of stress at various stages leading up to a jump; at the same time a sample of blood was withdrawn for subsequent analysis of its content of cortisol. The experiment was repeated on successive days. What was found, not surprisingly, was that the stress level increased to a maximum just before each jump; as training progressed, the magnitude of the change declined. What had not been anticipated was that the levels of blood cortisol matched both the increase in stress prior to a jump early on, and the lesser increase prior to a jump as training progressed. The development of techniques for measuring the content of cortisol and other hormones in saliva has obviated the need for taking blood samples, which is itself a mild inducer of stress in some people. By sampling the saliva of individuals assessed as less confident, cheerful, or sociable than others, the link between cortisol and stress has been confirmed. The same result was obtained when comparing individuals who complained of pains in the head and neck, or of disturbances in their digestive sysytem, with those who did not. Interestingly, increased cortisol was found only first thing in the morning, not during the rest of the day. This is in keeping with the effect of stress on sleep that was discussed above.

Another group of molecules that illustrate the link between mind and body are the enkephalins and endorphins. Both are peptides produced by breakdown of certain proteins in the brain (the enkephalins—from the Greek word *enképhalos* for brain—being only five amino acids long). The very discovery of enkephalins and endorphins attests to the fact that specific molecular changes underlie not just fear and apprehension, but mood and behavior also. The effects on the mind of opium—a mixture of compounds like morphine and heroin that are present in the seeds of the opium poppy *Papaver somniferum*—have been known since the time of the ancient Egyptians; the pain-relieving qualities of morphine have been exploited by doctors ever since. A hundred years ago the English physician Sir William Osler described morphine as "God's own medicine." Some two decades ago, it was found that morphine and other opiates bind to the plasma membrane of certain nerve cells. As a result of binding, the symptoms associated with their use, namely, euphoria, the relief of pain, and so forth, are transmitted in the brain. Since it seemed surprising that human nerve cells should contain receptors for plant-derived molecules such as the opiates, a search for similar molecules made in the body was initiated: The result was the discovery of enkephalins and endorphins by groups of scientists working in the United States and in Scotland. Although the molecular triggers leading to the synthesis of enkephalins and endorphins are not yet understood any better than the molecular consequences of their action like pain relief, euphoria, and so on, it is only a matter of time before this is achieved.

On the other hand, the action of enkephalins in stimulating the kind of fluid movement in the intestine that was referred to earlier, has been established. This link between a neurotransmitter and a body function such as fluid movement in the intestine is no longer surprising. Just as enkephalins act as neurotransmitters in the brain and as hormones in the rest of the body, so hormones like histamine or cholecystokinin that control bowel movement, act as neurotransmitters in the brain. Molecules of the immune system, like cytokines, likewise play a dual role: They stimulate B and T lymphocytes in the blood, but they also cause the release of ACTH from the brain, which as mentioned earlier is a hormone elevated in times of stress. Cytokines therefore account in part for the link between the immune system and stress. In short, there is no distinction between molecules of the endocrine system, the nervous system, and the immune system. In all cases a molecule elicits a response because it becomes attached to a receptor—a protein with a specific binding region—situated on the surface (spanning the plasma membrane) of a cell. The cell responds in whatever way it is programmed to do, be it liver, nerve, or lymphocyte. If the molecules involved in the processes of our mind are the same as those involved in the rest of our body functions, how can the distinction between mind and matter, between mental and physical stress, between "psychosomatic" and "physical" illness, be retained? It cannot.

How do the molecules that are produced by stress—epinephrine, cortisol, enkephalins, and endorphins—initiate diseases like peptic ulcer, cancer, or a heart attack? First of all, they do not do so on their own: They are but another risk factor toward disease, like our genes and other environmental factors such as nutrition, microbial infection, or pollution (see Table 2 in Chapter 4). In the case of peptic (stomach) ulcer, for example, we now know that an invading bacterium—*Helicobacter pylori*—which enjoys living in an acid environment like that of the stomach (into which we secrete 2 liters of hydrochloric acid per day), is a major contributory factor, as well as stress. The impact that nutritional status has on heart disease, or that ionizing radiations and certain viruses have on cancer, has already been mentioned. The important point to make is that the interplay between molecules like epinephrine and cortisol, enkephalins and endorphins, cytokines and other molecules (virtually every hormone so far discovered seems to be involved in one way or another in stress) is so complicated that it is not possible at present to construct a logical sequence of molecular changes leading to one or other disease. This is particularly true of cancer. In the case of heart disease, at least some of the events that lead up to it in a nonstressed person, such as the formation of atheromatous plaques in arteries, arrhythmias in heartbeat, lack of muscular exercise, and so on, are becoming fairly well understood. In the case of cancer, this is not yet so. This is one of the reasons why the link between stress and cancer is much more tenuous than that between stress and heart disease. What is becoming clear is that the initial molecular changes described herein appear to represent the body's attempt to ameliorate and to reverse the effects of stress: The action of epinephrine and cortisol, as well as of increased glucose uptake, in providing the tissues with more energy, is one example; the action of enkephalins and endorphins in countering pain, insomnia, and anxiety is another. In short, disease results when the beneficial action of these changes is overcome by the continuation of stressful stimuli. It is again a situation where controlled molecular changes redress a particular insult to the body, but where incessant insults lead to disease.

What kinds of drugs are available for treating the main kinds of stress like anxiety, depression, insomnia, and mild pain? It has to be said at the outset that in none of these ailments is the molecular basis fully known, so rational therapy is difficult and the drugs that are used are prescribed on the basis of a hit-or-miss approach, i.e., of clinical experience of efficacy. On the contrary, what knowledge we do possess about the molecular basis of anxiety or depression is based largely on pharmacological knowledge of how some antianxiety and antidepressive drugs work.

The most effective drugs used to treat anxiety are sedatives like the barbiturates and the benzodiazepines. A sedative is defined as a drug that has a calming effect, but it should be appreciated that at higher doses a sedative may also have a hypnotic effect, that is, it may cause drowsiness and sleep; at even higher doses such drugs may lead to anesthesia and coma. No drug is safe if taken in excess. The most common barbiturates are amobarbital (Amytal), pentobarbital (Nembutal), phenobarbital (Luminal), and secobarbital (Seconal). Barbiturates are rather powerful drugs with a number of side effects and their continued use leads to addiction. For these reasons they have been superseded for treating mild anxiety by the benzodiazepines. The most commonly prescribed of these are alprazolam (Xanax), lorazepam (Ativan), diazepam (Valium), and chlordiazepoxide (Librium). Though these drugs are certainly not without *some* side effects—no drug is—they are now among *the* most frequently prescribed of all drugs in the pharmaceutical business.

Barbiturates and benzodiazepines act in the same way, which is by potentiating the action of the neurotransmitter gamma-aminobutyric acid (or GABA) in the brain. The action of neurotransmitters is considered in detail in Chapter 8. For now, the point to note is that whereas the action of most neurotransmitters is to open ion channels and thereby transmit a nerve impulse, the action of GABA is the opposite: to inhibit the opening of ion channels and the transmission of nerve impulses. Barbiturates and benzodiazepines therefore cause inhibition of nerve impulses, which is compatible with their calming, antianxiety effects.

Although addiction to benzodiazepines is less than to barbiturates, it is not negligible and people do become reliant on them after many months of use. Half a million people in the United Kingdom alone are addicted to tranquilizers of one sort or another. The distinction between addiction and reliance or habituation is rather academic: What matters is whether someone finds it relatively easy to stop taking a drug or not, and—as with everything else to do with stress—there is an enormous person-to-person variation. It might be argued that diabetics takes insulin for life (if their diabetes is of the insulin-dependent type I), so why should a stressed, anxious person not take Valium for the same period? The analogy is false in that insulin is a normal constituent of the body (whose synthesis is impaired in insulin-dependent diabetics), whereas Valium is not. Continued use of *any* drug throughout life is undesirable, and the anxious, stressed person is better off trying to change his or her lifestyle, and to try to find alternative ways of reducing stress, if at all possible. The wives of the unemployed poor of Ireland or Spain a century ago probably survived better than their menfolk for the following reason—despite the fact that they gave the last scraps of food to their husbands: The women tended to turn to religion, the men to drink. Religious belief and prayer—the contemplative life in general—is entirely without harm, and those who are able to practice it are the lucky ones.

One in ten of us becomes clinically depressed at some stage of our lives; the most common cause is stress. The drugs used to treat depression fall into several classes. All work by essentially the same principle, which is to prolong the activity of certain neurotransmitters, in particular norepinephrine (a derivative of epinephrine) and serotonin. In that sense their action is opposite that of the barbiturates and benzodiazepines, which is to promote the inhibition of neurotransmitter action (in this case through GABA). Since depression is essentially a dampening down of nervous impulses, whereas anxiety is a heightening of nervous impulses (so that, for example, one's nerves are not relaxed enough to go to sleep), it is not surprising that antidepressants work by stimulating nerves whereas antianxiety drugs work by suppressing them. The drugs known as tricyclics (to reflect their molecular structure) prolong the action of both norepinephrine and serotonin, by preventing their removal from their site of action. They were originally developed as antihistamines (to alleviate, among other things, motion sickness), but proved to be more efficacious as antidepressants; an earlier chapter referred to the fact that several drugs were originally developed to cure one disease, but were fortuitously found to ameliorate another. For this reason, of course, the effects of tricyclics are not restricted to alleviating depression; a depressed person taking a tricyclic will probably fare quite well on a choppy sea. Amitriptyline (Elavil) and imipramine (Tofranil) are commonly prescribed tricyclics.

Drugs with a slightly different structure but similar mechanism of action are the heterocyclics, of which buproprion (Wellbutrin) is a good example. Another class of antidepressant drugs are the monoamine oxidase inhibitors like isocarboxazid (Marplan). This group of drugs boosts the action of norepinephrine and serotonin (both monoamines) by preventing their breakdown. Finally there is a group that acts specifically on serotonin by preventing its removal from the site of its action. Such drugs are known as selective serotonin reuptake inhibitors. Fluoxetine (Prozac) is the most-prescribed drug of this group of compounds. Its relative lack of toxic side effects is rapidly making it one of the favorite antidepressants in the field.

For the very seriously, clinically depressed patient, for whom no drug seems to work, there is always—as a last resort—electroconvulsive therapy (ECT), in which electric shocks are passed through the brain. Since each of our thoughts is in essence an electric current, the procedure is no more than what goes on in our brain anyway, except that we don't normally twitch and shudder when we think of ice cream, the clouds in the sky, or tomorrow's interview at the bank. Although the electrodes in ECT are positioned as precisely as possible over particular areas of the brain, it is still pretty much a hit-or-miss procedure. Nevertheless ECT has remarkably restorative effects on the seriously depressed and, now that the procedure is carried out under complete anesthesia, the patient feels no pain. The simultaneous administration of muscle relaxants also stops the convulsions.

Among the many people who suffer from depression there are those who are depressed on some days, but experience the opposite emotion—elation—on others. In its extreme form this manifests itself as mania, and the condition is referred to as manic-depression or bipolar affective disorder. Strictly speaking this is not so much a stress-related condition as one with a strong hereditary component, but since this book has been emphasizing the strong interplay between environmental and genetic factors as a cause of disease, it will be convenient to deal with it here. It goes without saying that we all have our good days and our bad: Life is a series of ups and downs, of feeling somewhat elated one day and slightly depressed the next. What distinguishes a manic-depressive is the intensity of this shift in mood: mania to the point of believing oneself to be richer or cleverer than is the case—to the point of chartering a jumbo jet to take some friends on holiday or of writing to the Nobel committee to complain why one has not been nominated for the prize; depression to the point of believing oneself to be persecuted by secret enemies and ultimately to the point of committing suicide. It is a feature of manic-depression that the periods of mania and depression are quite regular, each lasting some weeks or even months. Such oscillations in behavior suggest a derangement of some normal cyclic process, but what this is we do not know. Fortunately for manic-depressives there is a drug that dampens these oscillations, virtually reducing the intensity of the highs and lows to those of an average person. The drug is lithium carbonate, a simple inorganic salt similar to sodium carbonate (baking powder or soda). The active part is the lithium, not the carbonate. Lithium carbonate is fairly innocuous and in principle can be taken for life in small doses; however, there are numerous untoward interactions with other drugs (many because of its similarity to sodium) and its use should be minimized during pregnancy and lactation. On the other hand, it can be extremely efficacious, as illustrated in Figure 53. How does lithium work? Lithium has not been identified as an essential nutrient like calcium or zinc, so its action in alleviating the symptoms of manic-depression cannot be ascribed to restoring an apparent deficiency of lithium in the diet. Despite its wide use, the mechanism by which lithium acts is still unclear. It appears to inhibit one of the signaling mechanisms inside brain cells that is set in motion by stimulation of an enzyme in the plasma membrane of such cells by norepinephrine, but the details have to be worked out. So far as one can tell, there are virtually no direct toxic side effects to the use of lithium.

This discussion has summarized some of the medications that are on hand for those who suffer from the more severe man-

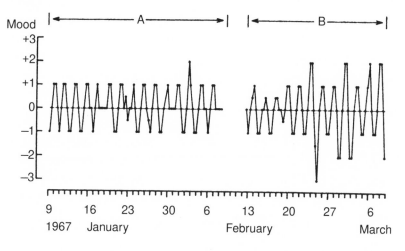

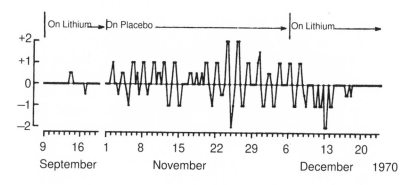

53. Efficacy of lithium. The diagram on the top shows the swings in mood, on a day-by-day basis, of a patient. The consistency of the swings in mood between mania and depression every 24 hours is remarkable. During the period marked A the patient was receiving a low sodium chloride intake (4.5 g/24 h, by mouth). During B he received a high sodium chloride intake (16.5 g/24 h). The diagram on the bottom shows what happened when the patient was receiving lithium carbonate (500 mg twice daily). The mood swings have all but disappeared. When lithium carbonate was discontinued and replaced by a placebo, the mood swings immediately returned, with the same periodicity. As soon as lithium carbonate (500 mg twice daily) was given again, the mood swings decreased and were virtually absent within 10 days. The patient remained in normal mood so long as he received lithium. When on lithium, he was able to carry out normal employment. Before lithium treatment his behavior was so disruptive that he was unemployable. From N. J. Birch in *Inorganic Perspectives in Biology and Medicine*, **1**, 173, 1978, with permission.

ifestations of stress. What of other treatments, especially those that may prevent the symptoms of stress from ever appearing in the first place? Not considered here are the obvious strategies of changing one's lifestyle, of taking regular exercise, and of maintaining a healthy diet (obesity, as well as anorexia and bulemia, incur both physical and mental stress), but rather some of the less well-defined therapies like psychoanalysis and religious practice, meditation and prayer. Some, like meditation, fall into the category of alternative medicine; some, like psychoanalysis, into that of orthodox medicine; and some, like religious practice and prayer, are not considered medicine at all, except by Christian Scientists. The message is straightforward: All of these therapies reduce stress because they calm the mind through a series of molecular changes that are similar to those brought about by barbiturates and benzodiazepines, by tricyclics and heterocyclics, by monoamine oxidase inhibitors and serotonin uptake inhibitors, and by lithium. If at this moment scientists are unable to identify the underlying molecular events, it is only a matter of time before this will become feasible.

The concept that Sigmund Freud (Figure 54) originally proposed is that by trying to recount our dreams, the hidden pressures in the mind that are responsible for initiating those dreams and that are the cause of certain types of aberrant behavior, are relieved. The therapeutic process depends acutely on conversation between the subject and the physician, who analyzes the dreams and our responses to certain questions; hence, analyst is a rather better term than shrink. Nowadays the emphasis has shifted from dreams to recalling past events in one's life, especially one's early childhood; this was well appreciated by Freud himself. While the therapeutic effects of any kind of cross talk are not in doubt, modern psychotherapy focuses more on the future than on the past. By talking about our current problems, and discussing possible approaches to solving life's difficulties, we are able to ameliorate their consequences.

The process of communicating our problems, especially our feelings of guilt, however, go back two millennia before Freud. The act of confessing one's sins in public is an integral part of the Christian religion, and public prayer goes back to Judaism. It has

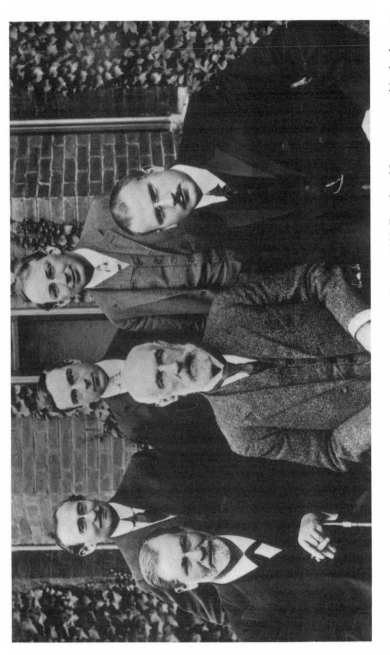

54. Sigmund Freud and Carl Jung. A group of early psychiatrists in Vienna, 1909. Freud and Jung are seated in the front row. Freud is on the left of the photograph, Jung on the right. Courtesy of The Wellcome Institute Library, London.

been retained in Christianity and has passed into the religion of Islam as well: It appears to be an essential ingredient of every organized form of worship that has emerged so far. It is likely that the beneficial effects were appreciated, albeit subconsciously, at the outset which is why this aspect has survived as a common feature of the great religions of the world. It is the author's view—though this is not the place to expand on it—that organized religions in general, including those of China, India, Egypt, Greece, and Rome, are as basic a feature of civilization as the emergence of scripts, coinage, or the creation of artifacts, because of their therapeutic potential. The findings of a group of neuroscientists from the University of California at San Diego seem to confirm this view: "There may be dedicated neural machinery in the temporal lobe concerned with religion. This may have evolved to impose order and stability on society," according to the head of the research team, Dr. Vilayanur Ramachandran. And if Judaism is therapeutic for the Jew, Buddhism for the Buddhist, Hinduism for the Hindu, Christianity for the Christian, and Islam for the Muslim, does this not suggest that each religion is largely in the mind of the individual? Did not Karl Marx call religion "the opium of the people"? Whatever one's belief, the conclusion that religion is predominantly in the mind of an individual does not, of course, in any way deny the erstwhile existence of holy men like Moses, Buddha, Jesus Christ, or Mohammed.

Prayer is only a part of the religious process. The thought that God's hand controls thunderstorms and lightning, floods and droughts, must have lessened the fright that these events gave to early man. And a belief in some form of afterlife contributes to the peace of mind of many of the sick and elderly and their families to this day. Nowhere, perhaps, is the analogy of conversation between patient and psychotherapist closer than in that between penitent and confessor in the Catholic Church. In each case the patient or penitent derives calmness of mind—relaxation as opposed to stress—as a result of talking about his problems with a second person; the fact that feelings of ambition and frustration, of desire and guilt, are given moral values in religions like the Christian faith is in a sense irrelevant to the healing process. In principle such two-way conversations should work between partners in marriage or in an equivalent relationship; in practice they do not because neither of the partners has the detachment and objectivity of a psychotherapist or priest. Nor, of course, do they work if the patient has no respect for the intellectual ability of the psychotherapist, or if the penitent is at heart a nonbeliever; in each case some measure of belief in the exercise has to be present.

A conversation between subject and listener need not be in private: For some people it works as well in public, as seen in the popularity of group therapy on the one hand and that of public confessions in church on the other. But is a listener required at all? It would seem not. In yoga, Zen Buddhism, meditation, or private prayer, the same results can be achieved on one's own. Prayer in the Judeo-Christian-Muslim religions, it may be argued, is intermediate between thinking one's own thoughts and speaking to another person, in the sense that it involves a conversation with God. Along similar lines, the reader must appreciate that the benefits of prayer insofar as the recipient of one's thoughts is concerned—be it one's dying mother or a starving child in Africa, the powers that decide on success or failure in one's forthcoming examination, or the elements responsible for bringing rain in times of drought—are beyond the scope of this book. Nevertheless the reader may like to note that a study financed by the John Templeton Foundation is about to be carried out on the efficacy of prayer on the recipient—the one prayed for: 600 patients about to undergo coronary artery bypass operations in various U.S. hospitals will be prayed for by a group of believers; another 600 about to undergo the same operation will not be prayed for. This study—never mind its outcome—illustrates the extent to which the benefit of prayer is accepted even in today's world. I shall not here discuss such concepts as an afterlife, or belief in God insofar as God is concerned, pausing merely to remind the reader of Einstein's words: "Religion without science is blind. Science without religion is lame." Nor can this discussion encompass such matters as miracles or extrasensory perception. The present work deals only with molecular changes within our own body that can be, and in many cases have been, measured.

There is no reason to suppose that yoga, Zen Buddhism, meditation, or private prayer are not as effective as the two-way processes discussed above in reducing mental stress and its risk to health. Indeed, regular transcendental meditation (TM) is said to reduce the number of hospital visits—inpatient or outpatient—in the United States by over 50% (these startling figures refer to patients registered with a special insurance group that runs TM programs, compared with patients registered with other insurance groups, and are provided by the company that runs the TM programs, so some caution in their accuracy is warranted). Many other forms of private thought or worship could be cited; I mention those particular four only because they are practiced by a very large number of people today, which in itself is an indication of their efficacy. All have in common two requisites: a stillness of mind and of body. You cannot meditate while listening to the news or watching the television monitor for details of your impending flight; you cannot pray while running to catch a bus or participating in a barn dance or eightsome reel. It is no accident that religious practices and yoga prescribe positions of the body that are associated with lack of movement, such as kneeling or sitting cross-legged. It is true that one can meditate or pray while lying in bed, but difficult if the bed is in a barrack room or adjacent to a disco. Why is it that yoga, Zen Buddhism, and other Eastern practices are so popular in the West today? It is, I suspect, because the element of stillness is an essential ingredient. While stillness and the contemplative life were the norms for the devout Jew, Christian, or Muslim in the thirteenth century, today this seems to be no longer true (though it has probably survived better in the Hindu and Buddhist religions). Witness the clapping of hands and the chanting of hymns set to jazz in many of our churches, or the bidding to prayer in mosques by ever louder calls from powerful radio transmitters. Those who believe that much of the stress of modern life is associated with noise and movement, turn intuitively to quietude and stillness as an antidote. This trend is particularly well illustrated by the growing popularity of Zen Buddhism (a form of Buddhism). Recall that Buddha was an Indian prince living around 2500 years ago. Going about his business he observed the suffering of life and death around him. He stopped being a worldly prince and became a simple man. As a result he received enlightenment. The essence of Buddhism is that we can all receive enlightenment if we follow in Buddha's footsteps and forget the ritual and formalities around us. Buddhism has no set beliefs, but it does reject the "logic" of Western ideas.

In 1934 Carl Jung (Figure 54), distinguished follower of Freud and exponent of the emerging practice of psychotherapy, wrote, "Great as is the value of Zen Buddhism . . . its use among Western people is very improbable." He would be surprised to see the number of people—young as well as old—who practice this and similar religions emanating from the East today. The fact that the mysticism of the Oriental mind is difficult to reconcile with the logic of the West as exemplified by our use of mobile telephones and digital watches, computers and e-mail through the Internet, has proved less of an obstacle than anticipated, whereas the qualities associated with the Oriental life—quiet, calm, silent, undisturbable—have become the goals of an ever-increasing number of people. Zen Buddhism is not a religion, having more in common with simple meditation: It is Buddhism without its religion, though it retains the Buddhist ideal of attaining satori, a kind of enlightenment. Listen to Kaiten Nukarila writing about satori in 1913: "Then our minds go through an entire revolution. We are no more troubled by anger and hatred, no more bitten by envy and ambition, no more stung by sorrow and chagrin, no more overwhelmed by melancholy and despair." Are not these the very qualities that were listed at the outset of this chapter as the main contributing factors to stress?

Before closing this discussion of preventing—and if necessary treating—stress by therapies without drugs, the reader is reminded that just as no two individuals are alike in their response to diet or to a microbial infection, so they are not alike in the workings of their mind either. While for one psychotherapy works best to combat stress, for another it is meditation or prayer, listening to Beethoven or blues, or merely crocheting a pattern, going for a walk or tending the garden; for many it is a combination of these ingredients. Each achieves a way of replacing anxiety or depression, insomnia or even pain, by a single

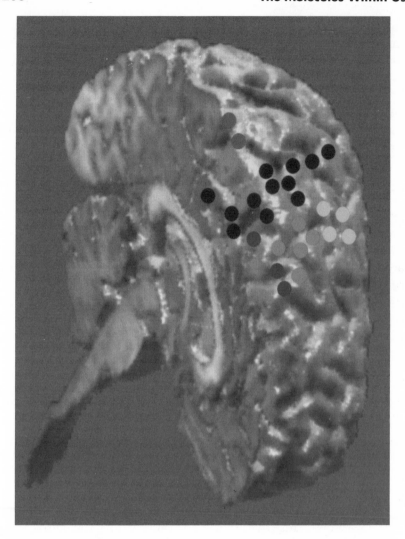

55. The laughter center in the brain. MRI (see Figure 58 on p. 227) reconstruction of one side of the brain (the cortical surface of the left frontal lobe) of a 16-year-old girl. Parts of the brain were stimulated with electrodes inside the skull to locate the focus of her intractable seizures. The five circles shaded light gray just underneath the black circles indicate an area of about 2 cm × 2 cm that consistently produced laughter when stimulated. At low stimulation the patient smiled; at higher stimulation she broke into a robust laughter. The other circles indicate areas that produced different responses. From an article by I. Fried, C. L. Wilson, K. A. MacDonald, and E. J. Behnke in *Nature,* **391**, 650, 1998, with permission.

quality: serenity leading to calmness of mind. Laughter is also immensely beneficial. Some scientists say that a minute's laughter is equal to 10 minutes aerobic exercise; at the same time the levels of "stress" hormones are reduced: Both cortisol and epinephrine were reduced in volunteers shown amusing videos. In support of these results, a recent report even claims to have located the "laughter center" in the brain (Figure 55). For those of us who accept these simple remedies, relief from stress is at hand.

The conclusion to be reached is the following: Stress, like the breathing of oxygen, the drinking of water, and the eating of food, is part of our daily lives. Mild stress like the excitement of achievement or falling in love, as well as that of jogging, a game of tennis, or a long hike, can be beneficial. Excessive stress is detrimental and leads to disease. My aim has been to illustrate some of the molecular changes that underlie stress and to summarize some of the treatments by which stress can be overcome.

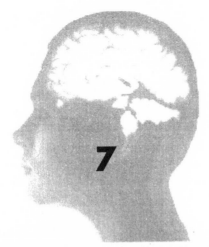

7

ORTHODOX VERSUS
ALTERNATIVE MEDICINE

hysicians, who have often spent more than a fifth of their working life in training, are naturally jealous of those who have spent half that or none at all in higher education, yet who presume to treat disease as effectively as they. Besides, the physician knows the location of every fiber in the body and can trace the path by which sensory impulses of sight, smell, hearing, taste and touch are transmitted through nerves to the muscles or to the brain. If as this century closes, physicians do not yet understand the molecular mechanisms involved in sorrow, anger, elation, or despair, neither do faith healers, acupuncturists, or homeopathic practioners. The nontraditional therapist is naturally resentful of the professional, when his own type of treatment yields the same, or an even better, result than that of the trained physician. The term nontraditional is used merely to distinguish such practitioners from trained physicians; within his own field, the trained acupuncturist is, of course, as professional as any surgeon, even if his methods by Western standards are not wholly accepted. Such rivalries between professionals and nontraditional practitioners or amateurs have existed for centuries, and are not confined to medicine. What professional artist or writer does not feel jealousy when a picture painted by an amateur like Winston Churchill is rated better than his own, or when a retired politician writes a bestseller? Conversely, what amateur biologist, like Charles Darwin, does not feel irritation when his ideas are rejected by the professional establishment of the day?

The conflict between professional and nontraditional in medicine goes deeper than mere personalities. It is the difference between orthodox and alternative medicine that is at stake. Orthodox medicine is assumed to be based on a rational approach, whereas alternative medicine seems to rest on a mixture of trial and error, dogma, dubious conviction, or worse. Yet, as we shall see, what is rational today may have seemed irrational yesterday, and vice versa. The orthodox medicine of the early 1800s, when homeopathy was being expounded as an alternative, consisted of purges, bloodletting, use of leeches, induced vomiting, high doses of mercury, and so forth. Today such treatments are considered unorthodox to say the least, if not harmful. Yet half of the drugs in use today are prescribed without detailed knowledge of their mechanism of action. We have referred several times to instances of drugs that were prescribed for one condition, which were then found to be more effective against another. Even aspirin (acetylsalicylic acid), a simple molecule more widely used and for a longer time than any other drug, is efficacious in different conditions—painkiller, to reduce fever, to thin the blood against heart attacks, for example—for reasons that are still not always fully clear. Hence, there is little fundamental difference between orthodox and alternative treatments: The only criterion should be whether they work or not. Since the conditions that each attempts to treat are sometimes different, comparison is difficult. Where the ailment is the same, orthodox medicine generally has a higher rate of success, but it is never 100% successful, and no professional physician worth his salt will ever *guarantee* a cure. While the chances of curing bronchial pneumonia may be 100 or 1000 times greater with penicillin than with ginseng, the efficacy of acupuncture for treating the pain associated with shingles (postherpetic neuralgia) is at least as good as any analgesic currently in use. The fact that we do not understand the basis of a remedy does not mean that it is ineffective.

Why, then, do alternative—or better, complementary—treatments sometimes work as well as orthodox ones? The answer is simple: because the molecules involved are ultimately the same. Take postherpetic neuralgia (intense, debilitating pain at the site of a persistent herpesvirus infection). The pain associated with this condition is the result of excessive impulses emanating from sensory nerve cells that have become infected with the chickenpox virus, a herpesvirus known as varicella zoster. Impulses are related to the opening of channels in the plasma membrane surrounding these nerve cells, channels that allow sodium ions to enter. Like other ion channels responsible for nerve conduction, the channels are proteins. Exactly what triggers their opening in virus-infected cells is not clear, though the openings markedly resemble those caused by the administration of capsaicin—the hot ingredient of chili peppers—and other pain-promoting substances. The result of an increased sodium ion concentration within the cells prompts the firing of nerve impulses to centers in the brain that experience the impulses as pain. Exactly how aspirin and other more potent analgesics (painkillers) act to inhibit these impulses is not fully understood, but it is likely that acupuncture achieves the same effect through the release of endorphins that, in turn, act at the same site as analgesics. In other words, both approaches go after the same molecular target—the pain-sensing cells in the brain.

I have already hinted that yesterday's orthodox medicine may become today's alternative therapy. More often, yesterday's alternative treatment is today's orthodox medicine. There are thousands of examples of treatments that were once viewed as an alternative, folk medicines for instance, that have found their way into the pharmacopoeia of today. Extract of foxgloves was once a remedy for people suffering from a heart condition. Today its active ingredient, digitalis, is the recommended treatment of choice for certain types of heart failure: It promotes the entry of calcium into the cells of the heart where it reactivates weakened muscle fibers.

For over 300 years, the bark of the cinchona tree has been used by South American Indians to combat malaria. Today, its active ingredient, quinine, and more potent chemically synthesized derivatives such as primaquine and chloroquine are prescribed for travelers entering malaria-infested regions. Unfortunately, malarial parasites, similarly to bacteria, become resistant to these drugs, and newer molecules are ever being synthesized to hit resistant parasites. Even quinine itself is once more being prescribed in certain cases where a patient has succumbed to chloroquine-resistant parasites. A combination of different antimalarial compounds is preferable to a single one for two reasons. First, because the two main pathogenic strains of the *Plasmodium* parasite, namely, *falciparum* and *vivax*, have different sensitivities against different molecules. Second, because a mixture of antimalarials is less likely to lead to the emergence of resistant strains than a single one: If strains resistant to one of the antimalarials emerge, they will still be sensitive to the second drug. Thus, artemisinin, a Chinese remedy that has been isolated from wormwood for more than 2500 years, is being effectively used against chloroquine-resistant *P. falciparum* for the very reason that it contains a mixture of active compounds, and people are turning full circle, back to *less* purified extracts of cinchona bark because it is now realized that the bark contains several different quinine derivatives, whose combination is more effective than a single purified compound. The aim of developing a suitable vaccine to prevent the disease from taking hold in the millions of people infected with the parasite remains high on the list of internationally funded collaborative research projects.

Another indigenous Chinese tree has been used in the treatment of cancer. This is a species of Taxus or yew. The stem bark of the *Cephalotaxus* tree provides a number of compounds that have been used in combination therapy against acute myelocytic leukemia (a cancer of the white blood cells) with apparent success rates as high as 50%. Over 60 other compounds of the stem bark of *Taxus brevifolia*, which have potential activity against cancers like breast cancer and cancer of the ovaries, have been isolated. And finally to India, for the benefits of the neem tree. Its leaves have been used for an antiseptic hand cream and its seeds for ailments as diverse as headaches, indigestion, and cancer; extracts are even being used as a male contraceptive. The twigs of the tree have cleansing properties and are used for brushing teeth: an instant toothbrush for those lucky enough to have a neem tree in their garden. The major ingredients that endow the neem tree with these healing properties are a class of molecules termed saponins. It is only a question of time before the precise molecular structure of these and other ingredients are analyzed and find their way into the pharmacopoeia of orthodox medicine. Such reasons make it important to preserve indigenous species, such as are found in the tropical rain forests of the world. To lose the possibility of exploiting these for potentially lifesaving drugs would be foolish indeed. We should not ignore our own plants. There is a tiny weed called *Arabidopsis thaliana* that is widespread throughout the northern hemisphere. Scientists have recently mapped the entire sequence of its five chromosomes, as a model for more than 250,000 species of plants. Several of the genes found in *Arabidopsis* appear to be involved in defense against disease. Although diseases affecting plants are different from those to which human beings succumb, there are some overlaps. Both plants and animals suffer from viral infections, for example, and although the specific viruses are different, there may be defense molecules in plants that we can adapt for our own use.

We should not be surprised at the efficacy of many folk medicines. True, some of these involve what Western medicine now considers unacceptable procedures, like bleeding, purging, vomiting, and so forth. But other remedies do not. We should remember that whereas orthodox drug discovery relies on clinical trials involving hundreds of patients to test efficacy and toxic side effects, this is unnecessary in folk medicine. Thousands of years of experience partially substitute for hundreds of patients in clinical trials. What folk medicine would have survived over the millennia if it had not been found to be of some benefit or if its toxic effects had proved too great? This is why pharmaceutical companies are now so eager to exploit the fruits of folk medicine. It is much cheaper and faster to isolate the active ingredient of a long-tested remedy that has survived for centuries than it is to synthesize millions of potentially efficacious compounds and to have to screen each one. It is for this reason that international treaties—following on from the Rio conference on biodiversity in 1992—are being put in place to prevent the countries whence these remedies originate—and whose economies lag behind those of the developed countries— from losing out on potentially lucrative sources of income. And some of the tenets of folk medicine are so similar to what we have been expounding here that it does not behoove anyone to sneer at them. Take one of the principal texts of Ayurvedic medicine as practiced in India; "Without proper diet, medicines are of no use; with proper diet, medicines are of no need." Is this not the point made in an earlier chapter?

What role does homeopathy play in all of this? It was Samuel Hahnemann of Philadelphia who in the last century propounded the "law of similia," which has since become the working definition for the practice of homeopathy: a system of medical practice that treats a disease by the administration of minute doses of a remedy that would, in healthy persons, produce symptoms of the very disease being treated. Although homeopathy is viewed with some disfavor by physicians, its principles underlie much of molecular medicine. Two examples will suffice.

The first concerns the discovery of vaccines, the use of which was discussed in a previous chapter. Smallpox was a devastating disease until 1976 when a worldwide vaccination program mounted by WHO (World Health Organization, a subsidiary of the United Nations) succeeded in eradicating the last-known outbreak in Somalia. Until then, victims who survived with a pockmarked face were the lucky ones: The rest died. One of the earliest uses of vaccination—the administration of a small amount of the causative agent in order to prevent disease by a subsequent and much larger amount—was carried out by Lady Mary Wortley Montagu (1689–1762) in 1718. Living for a time in Constantinople (now Istanbul) where her husband was British ambassador, she was aware of the local practice of "variolation" or inhaling the pus of a pox-infected victim. The procedure, which had been known in China and India for hundreds of years, was used largely to preserve the beauty (and hence the value) of the Circassian maidens in the seraglios of Constantinople and Baghdad.

Lady Mary believed in the efficacy of variolation so much that she inoculated her 3-year-old son with the disease: He lived to a ripe age, though of course he might have done so anyway.

One of the first recorded *experiments* was carried out nearly a century later by Edward Jenner (Figure 56) in the village of Berkeley in Gloucestershire in England. Jenner was a country physician who, in the late 1790s, had become impressed by the assertion of a local milkmaid, Sarah Nelmes, that she and many like her rarely contracted smallpox because they worked with cows. Jenner interpreted this experience by assuming that milkmaids became infected with cowpox through their handling of diseased cows, and that cowpox is sufficiently similar to smallpox to render such people immune to a subsequent infection with smallpox. He therefore repeated the procedure carried out by Lady Mary Wortley Montagu—and it has to be said by several others prior to Jenner—and vaccinated a boy, one James Phipps. In Jenner's case he used not smallpox, but the pus from the cowpox-infected hand of Sarah Nelmes. The hide of a cow called Blossom, reputed to be the animal milked by Sarah Nelmes, today hangs in the library of St. Georges Medical School in London, in whose hospital Jenner had received his medical training. In contrast to previous cases, Jenner then deliberately inoculated the boy with a subsequent, larger dose, of smallpox: James Phipps survived. Although Jenner had been elected a Fellow of the Royal Society (for his observations on the behavior of cuckoos), that august body refused to publish his observations. He therefore wrote a pamphlet that he published at his own expense. The principle of vaccination (the word is derived from *vacca*, the Latin for "cow") is nowadays carried out not with live virus but with attenuated or inactivated viruses. As already mentioned, it has been extended to the prevention, if not the eradication, of polio, measles, and rubella (whooping cough), and has been extended to vaccines against such bacterial diseases as tuberculosis, cholera, and typhoid.

The other example concerns the action of vitamins and trace metals. Vitamins and trace metals are not merely beneficial to our well-being, they are essential. But whereas a small amount is beneficial, an excessive amount is sometimes toxic. Strictly speaking,

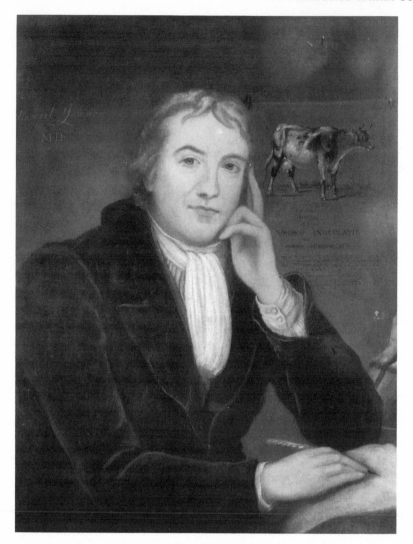

56. Edward Jenner. Oil painting (anon) with a cow in the background. Courtesy of The Wellcome Institute Library, London.

these are not examples of true homeopathic remedies, because the diseases against which vitamins and trace metals protect are not the same as those that result from an excessive intake. But if one allows a broader interpretation of homeopathy, vitamins and trace metals provide a good example of molecules that are beneficial in small doses, but toxic in large. Of course it could be argued that this is true of nutrition in general: A certain intake of glucose, fat, and protein is essential for the healthy body, whereas excess leads to obesity, heart attack, and stroke.

The complex manifestations of stress discussed in the previous chapter are in some ways an even better example, insofar as one particular form of stress, namely, mild exercise, benefits the heart by strengthening its muscles, whereas excessive exercise places too great a demand on those same muscles and leads to disease. These comments are made not to promote homeopathy, but because they illustrate a major, pretty self-evident, message of this book: A little of most things is good for you, too much is detrimental.

Vitamin A in small dietary amounts is essential for vision; it also prevents dry skin, respiratory infections, bone and tooth decay, and other problems. The role of vitamin A in vision is its most important one; it is also the one best understood in molecular terms, largely because of the elegant researches of the American scientist George Wald (Figure 57). The vitamin (also called retinol) is oxidized to a molecule containing two fewer hydrogen atoms, called retinal; this combines with a protein (opsin) to form rhodopsin, which is situated in a membrane within the retinal cells of our eyes. The properties of retinal are such that it is able to absorb visible light, rather like chlorophyll in plants. When it does so, rhodopsin undergoes a slight change of structure. As a result, the activity of several enzymes is stimulated and this leads, via a change in calcium ion concentration, to a nervous signal passing to the brain. In short, rhodopsin is an essential molecule that allows us to see.

In large doses vitamin A is toxic. The sickness developed by arctic explorers who ate polar bear liver has been ascribed to the latter's high content of vitamin A. The molecular mechanisms of toxicity are not clear. They do not impair vision, but may be related to a detrimental effect on those cellular membranes for whose development a small amount of vitamin A is necessary. If applied topically—to the skin—an oxidation product of retinal, namely, retinoic acid, is beneficial in rather high amounts against

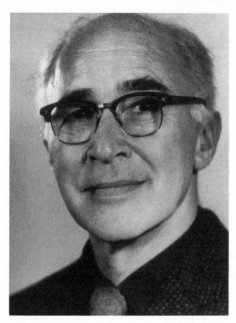

57. George Wald. Nobel laureate, 1967. He discovered the molecular mechanism by which retinal, a derivative of retinol (vitamin A), works in vision. Copyright: The Nobel Foundation, Stockholm.

skin complaints like acne, and is used as a skin cream. Of course most substances are more toxic when ingested than when applied topically, and are even more toxic when injected directly into the bloodstream.

Zinc, like all trace metals, is required in small amounts but is toxic in large; as with vitamin A, the mechanism of its beneficial effect is different from that of its toxicity. Zinc was chosen as an example because it is beneficial—in a third way—in intermediate amounts. We saw in an earlier chapter that total lack of zinc during parenteral nutrition leads to dry skin and other lesions; the same symptoms are displayed by people who lack a protein required for its absorption: The disease is a very rare one called acrodermatitis enteropathica. The relation of the disease to the action of zinc at the molecular level is not at all clear: All we know is that zinc is an integral part of proteins that control the transcription of DNA into RNA, and also plays a part in the catalytic action of certain enzymes. Additional zinc in the diet overcomes the lack of the specific absorptive mechanism in acrodermatitis enteropathica patients. Normally extra zinc is not required in the diet because the recommended daily intake of 15 mg is present in most foods anyway. The toxicity of zinc is greatest when it is inhaled as a vapor like that of zinc oxide, which is a hazard in the welding industry. Water-soluble salts of zinc are not nearly so toxic and can be ingested, according to the instructions on preparations sold in pharmacies, in amounts that are ten times higher than the recommended daily intake. It is in such intermediate doses that zinc plays a beneficial role.

All cells are surrounded by a thin membrane—the plasma membrane—that consists predominantly of two types of molecules: phospholipids and proteins. Phospholipids, it will be recalled, consist of water-soluble or water-loving (hydrophilic) and fat-soluble or water-hating (hydrophobic) parts. In membranes, the water-soluble parts are on the outside, making contact with water, and the fatty parts are in the middle, where they form a protective barrier against any water-soluble molecule, whether beneficial or toxic, from entering or leaving the cell. Beneficial molecules—nutrients like glucose, amino acids, and so forth—enter cells through pores made by specific proteins that are embedded in, and span, the phospholipid membrane. Other proteins form channels that specifically allow ions like K^+, Na^+, Ca^{2+}, and Cl^- to cross. It is such channels that form the basis for the passage of nerve impulses between the brain and the rest of the body, as described more fully in the next chapter. Some of the most toxic molecules that the body encounters are proteins secreted by infectious bacteria that give rise to cholera, diphtheria, tetanus, pneumonia, and staphylococcal infections. All of these proteins act on the plasma membrane of susceptible cells, and in several cases cause damage by puncturing holes in the membrane, just like the membrane-damaging proteins of the immune system. Zinc prevents such damage by literally closing the pores. It also appears to limit the spread of viruses like the common cold virus.

A strong proponent of zinc is George Eby of Austin, Texas. In the garage at the back of his house, Eby makes lozenges of zinc acetate, which is well absorbed and therefore more effective than other zinc salts sold commercially. He also recommends zinc ointment as a topical medicament. He should know. His daughter Karen was sunbathing in their garden when she was bitten on her navel by a black recluse spider, a creature whose venom is 100 times more poisonous than that of a rattlesnake. Rather than summon an ambulance, Eby calmly—well perhaps not so calmly—went to his garage, ground some of his lozenges into a paste with a little oil, and applied the mixture to the site of the bite, which by now was flaring up into a nasty wheal. Karen suffered no symptoms—apart from pain—and some days later the wheal turned into a scab and simply fell off. One isolated incident does not constitute a clinical trial (and perhaps the spider had lost some of its venom in a previous attack anyway) but there are sufficient cases of this kind, and of recovery from infections, that Eby and others have recorded. Although tall Texans are accused of telling tall tales, we should listen. Zinc ointment, after all, has been applied to infants' bottoms against microbial infections—"diaper rash"—for over 2000 years. Current studies suggest that zinc is also beneficial to the immune system and helps to prevent aging. Zinc lozenges taken against colds, sore throats, and mouth infections appear to work well for many people and zinc ointments applied topically against various bites and stings can also, as we have seen, be extremely effective. The reader will detect a certain diffidence in describing these beneficial effects of zinc. This is because its action is not nearly as potent as that of antibiotics or other drugs, which should remain the treatment of first choice; but since antibiotics are to be avoided wherever possible, because of the danger of resistant bacteria emerging, zinc exemplifies very well the concept of a complementary—rather than an orthodox—medicament. Of course, before trying any remedy, consult with your physician.

The modern followers of Samuel Hahnemann will wish to point to a second tenet of homeopathy that has not as yet been mentioned here. This is the "law of infinite dilutions," which states that the more a homeopathic remedy is diluted, the more effective it becomes. This is clearly not true of vaccines, vitamins, or any other molecule: When diluted too much, efficacy is lost because there are simply not enough molecules left to do the job. Adherents to the above "law" counter this by saying that the water used to dilute a homeopathic remedy somehow "remembers" the presence of the remedy, even when diluted so much that the chance of finding a molecule in a spoonful is less than 1 in 1000. The assertion that water "remembers" molecules in this way was repeated recently by an immunologist working in a French research establishment. The scientific journal *Nature* took the claim seriously enough to publish the findings that purported to support it. Following a howl of protest from its readers, *Nature* then sent a conjurer to the laboratory to see if some trick were involved: None could be found, but nor could the experiment be repeated elsewhere, and the claim eventually joined other contested observations like telepathy and UFOs. The claim was revived just at the time of writing this book, by the scientist concerned, Jacques Benveniste. He is suing three other French scientists (two of them Nobel laureates) for libel, because they have made statements to the French newspaper *Le Monde* to the effect that they considered the original observations rubbish (to put it mildly). The jury may be out as far as the libel case is concerned, but not in regard to the science. Stop press: Benveniste has lost his libel case, but only because the *tribunal de grande instance* dismissed the action: Benveniste had filed a civil suit; he should have filed a penal one.

Our explanation for the assertion that a spoonful containing less than a single molecule of a remedy may be efficacious, is that it reflects the "placebo" effect. This is the term given to a positive reaction when a patient receives—unknown to him—an innocuous substance like a sugared pill in place of a proven drug. The extent of the placebo effect is often extremely high: Over 50% of patients suffering from duodenal ulcer recover if given a placebo instead of a conventional drug (which again emphasizes the strong connection between the mind and the gut that was referred to in the previous chapter). The reason they do so is either because they would have recovered anyway (the body—unlike a malfunctioning automobile—has a remarkable capacity for self-recovery), or because they believe in the therapy so much that their "positive thinking" causes molecular changes that aid recovery.

The power of belief can be a very strong force, and may underlie many complementary treatments. These include the following; I am quoting directly from the brochure of treatments that are on offer at a typical Natural Health and Fitness Center in London, England. *Acupuncture,* a painless treatment that corrects the energy balance within a person by the insertion of fine needles at specific points on the skin; acupuncture has been found to enhance health and the immune system as well as addressing specific symptoms. *Alexander technique,* a course of lessons that enables one to become more aware of balance, posture, movement, and any tensions previously unnoticed. *Aromatherapy:* essential oils, extracted from plants, are applied to the body through massage, and are able to penetrate the body through the skin; oils are selected according to the needs of each individual, and can help with a wide range of problems. *Biodynamic massage;* by mobilizing the body, this massage helps to release blocked energy flow and chronic muscular tension, so reducing stress. *Chavutti Thirumal massage;* originating in India, this is a powerful full-body treatment where the therapist uses the feet to massage the body, which gives a much deeper pressure and is able to cover the full length of the body with each sweeping stroke. *Chinese herbs:* the use of plants for healing, to prevent illness and promote better health, treating the person as a whole. *Chinese medicine. Chua-Ka massage:* a very deep tissue massage emphasizing the connection between mind and body. *Decleor & Dr. Hauschka holistic skin care treatments. Feng Shui,* a system of looking at one's home or workplace in order to create harmonious surroundings by encouraging the smooth flow of "chi" or universal energy. *Healing. Homeopathy. Indian head massage:* massage of the scalp, face, and shoulders, which soothes, comforts, and rebalances the energy flow in order to promote a feeling of peace, tranquility, and well-being. *Manual lymphatic drainage,* an extremely light, repetitive, hands-on treatment that increases the movement of the lymphatic system of the body throwing its cleansing, regenerating, and healing powers into top gear. *McTimoney chiropractic,* a method devised to safely restore a patient's total structural integrity; chiropractors check and subtly adjust bones of the skull, thorax, spine, pelvis, and limbs. *Metamorphic technique:* a subtle technique that changes, transforms, and heals; using a light touch on the spinal reflexes in feet, hands, and head, thereby stimulating the recipient's own inner energies. *Optimum nutrition. Osteopathy/cranial osteopathy:* a very gentle technique in which the osteopath's highly trained sense of touch is used to identify and release tensions and disturbances within the musculoskeletal system, not only in the skull, but throughout the body. *Pilates;* this method improves muscle control, flexibility, strength, tone, and coordination; the matwork class is a series of interconnected movements integrating mind and body resulting in increased energy and relaxation. *Psychodynamic counseling,* which enables one to become aware of unconscious processes that are causing anxiety and pain; talking with the counselor in a supportive environment in order to discover ways of living a more satisfied and balanced life. *Psychotherapy:* the application of psychology in the treatment of disorders of a psychological nature; the treatment can use relaxation and imagery techniques in order to find the cause of the problem. *Reflexology,* a form of foot massage that has profound effects on the entire person; the feet are a map of the body and dysfunction in any area can be reflected there. *Reiki;* acting on the aura, physical and emotional levels, this is a system of healing using the cakras of the body. *Rejuvenessence facial massage:* a light massage treatment of the face, which releases muscular tension and gently helps the connective tissue to regain its elasticity and vitality, thereby reducing frowns, wrinkles, and worry lines and greatly improving complexion and texture of the skin. *Remedial massage. Shiatsu:* a body therapy using a combination of Japanese finger pressure and massage techniques; this works by stimulating the body's energy flow in order to promote good health. *Spineworks:* this nonforce technique assists in aligning the vertebrae and restoring the integrity of the spine; combining tendon and ligament releases, collulone point release, muscle balancing techniques, and remedial stretches, spineworks provides one with a gentle, powerful, and effective form of body treatment, facilitating the body's own innate sense of physical and emotional well-being. *Sports therapy and massage. T'ai Chi:* a martial art that began in China 1000 years ago; today, however, most people practice it to gain the great health benefits it has to offer. *Thai massage:* a dynamic and interactive form of massage that relaxes muscles and stimulates the lymph, blood, and energy flows; it works by mobilizing and opening the joints, gently stretching muscles and tendons. *Therapeutic massage. Tibetan massage and healing:* the technique of this finger pressure massage depends on the patient's energetic state and needs; the full body treatment emphasizes the balance of the five elements of air, fire, water, earth, and space. *Tu-ina massage:* related to acupuncture, whereby pressure is applied in varying degree to the body; Tu-ina removes blockages to the flow of energy, thus restoring balance, boosting the immune system, and alleviating many common ailments. *Yoga,* including yoga for pregnant and postnatal women. The treatments described give an excellent overview of the kind of complementary therapies that are available. Many rely on one or other form of massage. This was known even to the ancient Greeks: Compare the above descriptions of some of the treatments with the advice of Hippocrates 2400 years ago: "Physicians must be experienced in . . . rubbing that can bind a joint that is loose and a joint that is too hard." No physiotherapist treating a case of arthritis could disagree with that. Indeed, there is obviously much overlap between conventional and complementary medicine. But it must be reiterated that in severe diseases complementary medicine is no match for orthodox treatments. Even less successful is no treatment at all: Time and again we read of Christian Scientists who have refused treatment for ailments like blood poisoning or leukemia (often on behalf of their children); regrettably most of them die.

The wealth of the pharmaceutical industries is second only to that of the oil companies, and some spend up to 30% of their income on research and development; a major company like SmithKline Beecham spends 15%, which is probably a good average for the industry as a whole. The budget for the National Institutes of Health in Bethesda, Maryland, which is the main funding agency for medical research in the United States, is in excess of $10 billion per year, and medical charities like the Howard

Hughes Foundation contribute many millions more. How, we are entitled to ask, has this helped in the fight against disease, and what are the prospects for the future? Although I referred earlier to the disappointing lack of progress in regard to a cure for cancer, all is not doom and gloom even for this disease, and so far as heart disease, ailments of liver, kidney, and other organs are concerned, there have been some spectacular advances, not least in transplant surgery. The proof of the pudding is in the eating, or rather in the not eating, since the increased longevity of Americans owes much to a reduced caloric intake coupled to a greater awareness of the importance of exercise. The same is true of Western Europe, Japan, and other developed countries with good medical infrastructure.

In order to devise new treatments for disease in a rational manner, the molecular changes underlying the disease need to be understood. Where the disease is in the blood, as in anemia, this is fairly straightforward as it is a simple matter to take a blood sample and analyze it; even in this case, however, the *cause* of the disease is often elsewhere—for example in the bone marrow where the precursor cells of the red and white blood cells are made. But what of diseases of liver, kidney, heart, or brain? Although it is possible to take biopsy specimens from within an organ like the liver, this is difficult, dangerous, and provides only very small samples. Hence, much of what we know about the molecular changes that underlie diseases of these organs is limited to circumstantial knowledge gained from taking samples of blood, urine, and—in the case of brain—cerebrospinal fluid, itself an extremely painful process. It is just in this area—that of diagnosis—that some spectacular advances have been made over the last decade that show promise of achieving the ultimate goal: noninvasive diagnosis or direct analysis of molecules within our organs without having to remove bits from them. How did this advance come about? Through research not in biology but in the field of spectroscopy, which encompasses physics and chemistry.

The technique to which I refer is nuclear magnetic resonance or MR (magnetic resonance) for short. It had been known for many years that if molecules in a solution are subjected to high magnetic fields, some of their constituent atoms—or rather the nuclei within the atoms—will tend to align themselves according to the field; the underlying principle is the same as that by which the needle of a compass is attracted to the earth's magnetic center, near the North Pole. These polarized nuclei can be made to resonate, by absorbing some energy, if they are subjected to a pulse of radiofrequency radiation. If the applied radiofrequency field is then switched off, the nuclei relax back to their original, random positions. This gives out a weak signal. The frequency at which nuclei do this varies from atom to atom. Of the atoms present in organic molecules it is relatively easy to detect hydrogen and phosphorus, but nitrogen and carbon are more difficult to detect and oxygen even more so. Consider the example of methanol (CH_3OH): Because of interactions between neighboring atoms, the signal from the three H atoms on the C atom is different than that from the H atom on the O. By carefully analyzing such signals or spectra, the composition of a molecule can be deduced. Not just the composition, but the actual position of every atom in a molecule; one of the major feats of modern biochemistry has been the determination of the three-dimensional structure of proteins in the test tube, based solely on analysis of their constituent H atoms—several hundreds in even a small protein—by nuclear magnetic resonance.

Because the magnetic field and the signals that are returned penetrate the tissues of the body, one is able to detect molecules deep below the surface of the skin; by focusing the radiofrequency pulse on a particular area, at a particular depth, it is possible to obtain a spectrum from a slice of liver, kidney, heart, or brain. Heart presents some difficulties, because it is continually moving with the contractions of its muscles, but new techniques are being developed to allow for this. Because the concentration of most molecules within cells is rather low, the signals are weak, and therefore limited as yet to the most abundant molecules; but already it is possible, for example, to detect the level of lactic acid in brain (Figure 58)—indicative of a slight stroke—or that of ATP in muscle—indicative of healthy energy metabolism (Figure 59), and so forth. In the case of a cancer growing within the body it is possible to follow the effectiveness of certain therapies by analyzing some of the molecules that are typically present in cancer cells but not in the neighboring normal cells, and so on. The technique is still in its infancy, but we can expect exciting advances in the future.

What has just been described is sometimes referred to as MR spectroscopy or MRS to distinguish it from MR imaging or MRI (Figure 58). Imaging is much easier to perform and depends simply on measuring the H of H_2O; water, it will be recalled, makes up over 60% of most tissues and is therefore the most abundant molecule present. The image that is produced by MR is the opposite of that produced by X-ray imaging: Whereas X rays reveal hard tissues, namely, bone, MR reveals all of the soft, water-containing tissues, namely, the rest of the body. I have referred to MR as being noninvasive. X rays cannot be considered to be noninvasive as they are known to cause local damage—especially to DNA—and are therefore mutagenic, though not as strongly as ionizing radiations from radioactive fallout; nevertheless the use of X-ray imaging has been severely limited over the past few decades. Is not MR equally damaging, then? The answer is no. So far as we can tell at the present time, MR causes no adverse effect on the cells of the body at all: There is vitually no temperature rise and no ionization or other chemical change has ever been detected. Of course, skeptics of novel medical advances will retort with the comment that while current MR techniques may be genuinely noninvasive, this may not be true of future modifications involving more powerful magnets in order to increase the sensitivity of the method. To this one can only reply "wait and see." The fact is that at last we have a technique that has tremendous potential for analyzing molecular changes in diseased tissues and that is already being used to great advantage.

In general, of course, advances in new technologies are not so dramatic or fundamental; on the other hand, if a novel therapy saves but one life, or improves the well-being of only a handful, it is surely worth having. An example of a quite unspectacular advance, but one that has significantly prolonged life span in several types of leukemia, is that of rational combination therapy. Within a clone of continuously dividing cancer cells, there is the chance of an occasional mutant arising; if that cell has an advan-

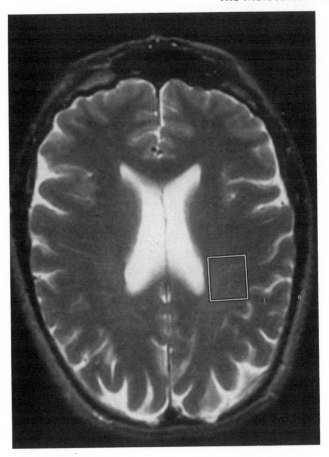

58. MRI and MRS of brain. (Left) An MRI (magnetic resonance imaging) scan of the writer's brain. (He volunteered to be a "control" in a study of brain function.) Successive slices of the brain at different depths were analyzed; a typical slice is shown. The brain appears to be normal. (Right) An MRS (magnetic resonance spectroscopy) scan of a section of the MRI scan analyzed by spectroscopy. The time required for spectroscopy is much longer than that required for imaging. For this joint MRI/MRS study, the subject had to lie absolutely still, with his head inside the magnet, for about an hour. A typical slice, corresponding to that analyzed by MRI on the left, is shown. The peaks indicate different molecules: mI is myoinositol (a residue of certain phospholipids); tCho is total choline derivatives (a residue of most phospholipids and the molecule from which the neurotransmitter acetylcholine is made); tCr is total creatine derivatives (see Figure 59); NAA is N-acetyl aspartate, a derivative of the amino acid aspartate that may act as a neurotransmitter. A high peak indicates

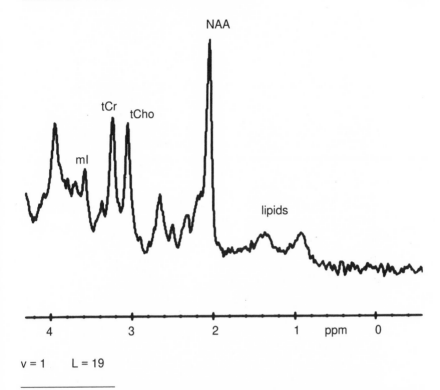

v = 1   L = 19

___

healthy neurons. Even better, from the writer's point of view, is the absence of any lactic acid peak: The presence of lactic acid indicates a mild stroke or other disorder. Images courtesy of Drs. Franklin Howe and John Griffiths, St. George's Hospital Medical School, London.

tage over all other cells by being able grow in the presence of a drug that would normally prevent its growth (i.e., by being resistant to the drug), it will outgrow all other cells, just like bacterial mutants that are resistant to the effect of an antibiotic. During the 1950s and 1960s many analogues of the constituents of DNA, namely, nucleotides, were synthesized in the hope that they might be useful as anticancer agents. An analogue in this context is a molecule whose structure resembles an ingredient of our body sufficiently to fool the enzyme that normally handles it: It binds the enzyme but is not changed by it, so causing inhibition of that pathway. Depending on precisely what part of the natural

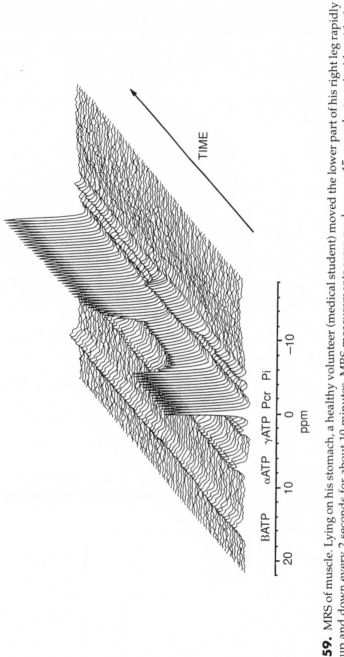

59. MRS of muscle. Lying on his stomach, a healthy volunteer (medical student) moved the lower part of his right leg rapidly up and down every 2 seconds for about 10 minutes. MRS measurements were made every 15 seconds, to coincide with the subject's breathing and with his leg being in the correct position in relation to the magnet. βATP, αATP, and γATP all refer to ATP (each molecule gives three distinct peaks, one for each of the three phosphate residues; see Figure 29 in Chapter 3); Pi is phosphate ion; PCr is phosphocreatine, a "high-energy" molecule like ATP, which keeps ATP levels topped up. It is seen that as exercise commences, PCr levels fall and Pi levels rise (with little change in ATP). As soon as exercise stops, PCr and Pi levels return. Spectra courtesy of Harry Rossiter and Dr. Brian Whipp (Physiology) and Drs. Franklin Howe and John Griffiths (Biochemistry), all at St. George's Hospital Medical School, London.

molecule is changed, the analogue may even be handled as normal by the first few enzymes of a pathway, and clog up the machinery only later on. This is how the anticancer drugs, two of which are illustrated in Figure 60, work. Because the changes in

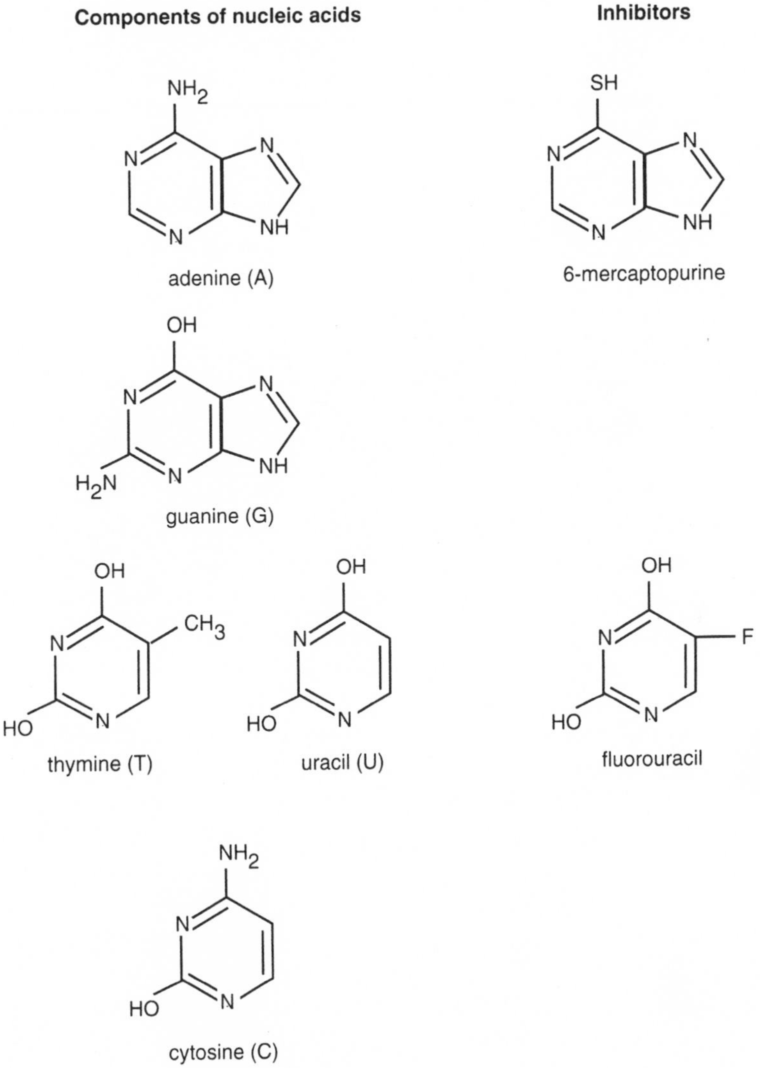

Components of nucleic acids   **Inhibitors**

adenine (A)

6-mercaptopurine

guanine (G)

thymine (T)   uracil (U)   fluorouracil

cytosine (C)

60. Nucleotides and some analogues.

the nitrogen (N)-containing rings allow the molecules to add a sugar residue, followed by a phosphate residue to form an intact nucleotide (N-containing ring linked to sugar linked to phosphate, as shown in Figure 29 in Chapter 3), they inhibit at the later stages of DNA synthesis. It was appreciated that there would be toxic side effects, since the drugs were not specifically targeted to cancer cells, and would therefore be toxic to all dividing cells. But apart from the bone marrow (the site of blood cell renewal) and the lining of the gastrointestinal tract (where cells are also constantly being renewed), there are not so many tissues of the body where active cell division, and therefore DNA synthesis, occurs. And if it is a question of the likely death of a person—often a child—a certain amount of toxic side effects is acceptable. What depressed clinicians in those days was the fact that to every analogue that was synthesized, a resistant mutant would eventually arise. Resistance arises, as with bacteria resistant to an antibiotic, through various causes; one is that cells overproduce the enzyme that is targeted to such an extent that the analogue is without effect. In other words the toxic effects of the analogue are simply bypassed. Rational chemotherapy seemed therefore not to provide the answer. Then, however, clinicians began to monitor carefully the leukemic cells that remained and aimed not for 100% eradication, but for something less: in other words to continue treatment with one drug for only a limited time, before resistant mutant cells emerge. At this point, treatment is switched to a different analogue, and so on. By this means some very encouraging results have been obtained, and life expectancies have increased to the point where—at least in the case of adults—the patients die of natural causes.

An approach that goes back even further than the nucleotide analogues just described is to use nitrogen mustards to destroy cancer cells. Such compounds were originally used as mustard gas to maim and kill soldiers in their trenches during World War I. Subsequently the toxicity of these molecules was recognized as causing the depletion of white blood cells from the circulation and from bone marrow. By 1942 the use of nitrogen mustards like cyclophosphamide was transferred from the war against people to the war against disease (they were not used during World War II).

This approach was pioneered by Louis Goodman and Alfred Gilman, two American pharmacologists who collaborated together at Yale over many years. They were so close, and had so much respect for each other, that Gilman gave his friend's name to his son; Alfred Goodman Gilman followed in the family tradition and became an eminent pharmacologist. Goodman and Gilman reasoned that if cyclophosphamide causes the loss of normal white cells, it might prove effective in killing cancerous white cells like a lymphoma. Their suspicion was confirmed, though they were probably unaware of it at the time. What happened was that an American ship carrying stocks of nitrogen mustard to Italy in January 1944 (as a retaliatory weapon in case it should be used by the enemy) was torpedoed during the attempt by the Allies to land on the beaches of Anzio. Some of the nitrogen mustard gas leaked out. Among those exposed to it was an American sailor who had cancer; to his surprise, his condition improved. Through Goodman and Gilman, then, the use of nitrogen mustards found its way into the cancer clinic, but of course toxicity is high. It is partly offset by the fact that molecules like phosphoamide derivatives are not themselves toxic, but only become so after conversion within cells to the active compounds: These cause damage predominantly through their interaction with DNA. Any drug that chemically modifies DNA is, of course, potentially mutagenic and might therefore *induce* cancer. In order to selectively *kill* cancer cells it is therefore important to get the dose exactly right, and to try to ensure that the drug—or more accurately the prodrug— reaches its target, namely, the cancer cells rather than other cells. This is a pretty tall order, and the use of molecules like phosphoamide over the past 50 years has declined because of their high toxicity (against dividing cells like those of bone marrow and the gastrointestinal tract). Just recently their application has been revived through novel derivatives that are specifically targeted toward cancer cells (the dream of all oncologists), because they are converted from prodrug to active drug in just those cells. The action of phosphoamides in killing white blood cells like lymphocytes has also been exploited in trying to suppress the immune system after an organ transplant; but, as might be anticipated, their use as immunosuppressants is limited because of their toxicity. The point we wish to stress yet again is that most therapy of disease by drugs is poised on a knife edge between successful cure and inadvertent damage elsewhere.

The main difficulty in treating cancer, then, is that the cells are so similar to the normal cells of our body. Hopes have been raised countless times, only to be dashed again, at reports of a molecule that is specific to cancer cells. Most of the time one finds only molecules that are *not* present, though they are in the cells from which the cancer is derived. This is because many types of cancer cell are nonspecific versions of the original cell: That is, cell-specific molecules like myosin of muscle cells, or immuno-globulin of lymphocytes, or hormones of endocrine cells, are lost. The reader is reminded that cancer is not a single disease, but a group of diseases, depending on the type of cell from which it is derived: Cancers arising from the cells (termed epithelial) that line the surfaces of our body and all of our organs, including the inside surfaces of organs like the gastrointestinal tract, are by far the most common and are called carcinomas; cancers arising from the white blood cells are leukemias and lymphomas, and cancers arising from muscle and connective tissue (cells beneath the epithelial layers and elsewhere) are called sarcomas. All are derived from multiplying cells and it is during the cell division cycle that things start to go wrong and cancer cells emerge. The absence of molecular markers—especially on the surface—of cancer cells is what has bedeviled attempts at rational approaches aimed at their destruction. Surgical removal of a solid mass of cancer cells—called a tumor—is of course feasible, but residual cancer cells are often left behind and it is impossible to remove all of the secondary tumors—the metastases—that arise when the cancer spreads to other tissues. The same is true of radiation treatment of tumors that are inaccessible to surgery. Yet did I not say that the T-lymphocyte system that destroys virus-infected cells also serves a general purpose of immune surveillance that includes cancer cells, and that might therefore be pepped up in some way to provide a novel approach? This is correct, and some initial successes have already been reported. The potential suc-cess of immunotherapy is not incompatible with the earlier state-ment concerning the lack of molecular markers on cancer cells.

For it will be recalled that the killer T cells recognize not a molecule on the surface of the doomed cell, but a small peptide that is derived by breakdown of a protein within the cell (see Figure 49 in Chapter 5).

An approach that overcomes the need to distinguish a cancer cell from a normal one is based on the fact that for a solid tumor to grow, individual cells need to be supplied with nutrients from the blood, just like all the other cells in the body. In short, a growing tumor needs to establish a blood supply for the cells inside the growing mass. The establishment of such a blood supply is known as angiogenesis, and recently two drugs that interfere with angiogenesis—at least in mice—have been discovered: they have been termed angiostatin and endostatin. Each molecule is part of a protein—plasminogen and collagen 18, respectively—that is a normal constituent of our tissues, but that has no effect on tumors. However, both the peptides, angiostatin and endostatin, have anticancer activity in that they are able to cause massive tumors in mice to shrink to virtually nothing. As soon as treatment is stopped, however, the tumors return and now spread to other sites as well. When angiostatin and endostatin were injected simultaneously, the result was staggering: not only did the tumors vanish, but they did not return when treatment was stopped. Because the blood vessels that supply a tumor with nutrients are made up of normal, not cancer, cells, inhibition of their growth does not lead to the emergence of resistant cells, as in the case of chemotherapy with nucleotide analogues that was mentioned earlier. Moreover, the treatment is good for *any* type of cancer, since all tumors are dependent on a blood supply. It even works against some leukemias (in mice) because angiogenesis in the bone marrow is involved in producing leukemic cells. In the words of Judah Folkman of Children's Hospital in Boston, who has been working on the relationship of angiogenesis to tumor growth for 30 years, ". . . if you have cancer and you are a mouse, we can take good care of you." So what are the prospects for treating people with angiostatin and endostatin? In principle, they are excellent; in practice, it is too early to say, for the simple reason that the two drugs have not yet been produced in sufficient quantity to test on people. Even as this sentence is being written, a company called Entremed—in collaboration with Bristol-Myers Squibb and others—is churning out angiostatin and endostatin in order to accumulate enough for human testing. Watch this space!

The potential advances associated with knowledge of what roles our genes play in common diseases like heart attack or stroke have already been alluded to. The payoff will be twofold. The first involves the gene in question, the second concerns the protein specified by the gene. In the case of a missing or faulty gene, it is in principle possible to supply the body with the correct gene, synthesized in the laboratory. The problems associated with introducing genes into specific cells, however, are enormous. The plasma membrane surrounding each of our cells is designed so as to keep such foreign material out—foreign in the sense that DNA is not present in the bloodstream and is not normally transferred from cell to cell. Ways of surmounting this include packaging the DNA inside a phospholipid vesicle (see Figure 13 in Chapter 2) that a cell may take up as though it were a vesicle surrounding a nutrient molecule like triglyceride, or attaching the DNA to an inactivated DNA virus that is able to enter a sensitive cell through the normal invading process. So far, the success of this type of gene therapy—applied to cystic fibrosis, for example—has been pretty limited, but these are early days. The potential of gene therapy, once the mode of delivery has been worked out better, is enormous, since the technique is not, of course, restricted to hereditary diseases like cystic fibrosis. Any disease in which a faulty gene is implicated, as in cancer, or a normal gene fails to function properly, as in neurological disorders like Parkinson's or Alzheimer's, in cardiovascular disorders like atherosclerosis or even in infectious disorders like AIDS (malfunctioning T lymphocytes) is a potential target. If successful treatment by gene therapy is still a few years away, there is no doubt that within a decade or two it will be as common as protein therapy—like insulin for diabetics or factor VIII therapy for hemophiliacs—is today.

In the case of a gene that is actively causing trouble—because it is being overexpressed or because it has become mutated—through the production, for example, of a protein that overrides the controls that limit cell division as in cancer, it is possible to inhibit the gene by introducing into the cell short stretches of chemically modified nucleotides that correspond to a part of the sequence ("antisense" nucleotides like AATGCCG... in place of TTACGGC...) and effectively "glue up" the function of the gene. This approach is at an even earlier stage of development.

Attacking the function of inappropriately expressed proteins has received a tremendous boost by being able to determine the precise three-dimensional structure of a protein through methods like MR spectroscopy (and X-ray crystallography). In the case of an enzyme, for example, it is possible to design molecules that will fit into the catalytic pocket as neatly as the molecule that normally does so, but that in this case remain bound to the enzyme and therefore inhibit its function. The use of computer graphics to develop such a "designer molecule" is illustrated in Figure 61. The enzyme is the neuraminidase of influenza virus. This is the N protein that was mentioned in relation to influenza epidemics in Chapter 5; the enzyme is essential for the infectivity of the virus. The designed molecule is called zanamivir and is now in clinical trials. Such inhibitory molecules have, in fact, been known for a long time: The analogues of nucleotides used in chemotherapy of cancer are one example. Another example is the volatile molecule DFP (diisopropylfluorophosphonate).

DFP causes paralysis of muscles via its inhibition of an enzyme that normally terminates the action of a neurotransmitter—in this case acetylcholine—in the way that the antidepressant inhibitors of the enzyme monoamine oxidase work (see the previous chapter). In this instance the effects are lethal. Aside from its use as a research tool to study the relevant enzyme (acetylcholinesterase), it found favor with military commanders: a derivative called *sarin* kills within 15 minutes of contact. The United States alone at one time had stockpiled sufficient quantities of the compound (appropriately called nerve gas) to annihilate every human being on the globe (targeted delivery, of course, would have been another matter). It was not used militarily by either side during the 1939–1945 conflict; its use to exterminate the inmates of concentration camps is another story. Since then, nerve gas has been used only once: by Iraq, during its war with Iran in the 1980s. The Iraqis attacked Majnoon Island, which had been taken from them by the Iranians. They bombed it with a cocktail of nerve gas, nitrogen mustard, and mycotoxins; whether anthrax was included is not clear. It was certainly the first time that chemical and biological weapons were used simultaneously. It was also the first time that the effects were well-documented, as UN experts were able to visit the site subsequently and to examine the survivors. The burns on the flesh of those exposed to the nitrogen mustard blister, open up and constitute a primary site for infectious microbes: Whether the victims became infected with anthrax sent in bombs or from the anthrax that was already on the ground (the island had been a military installation) is not known. The mycotoxins that were released from the bombs certainly played their part. Apart from skin burns, the survivors (many of course were killed outright) suffered from damage to eyes, lungs, and respiratory system. Iranian physicians who were tending the survivors were able to photograph the wounds firsthand. The writer can attest to the devastating consequences of this combination of chemical and biological warfare because the results were presented at a UNESCO conference on the Misuse of Biological Knowledge that he attended in 1997.

The design of molecules to fit into the pocket or groove of a protein is not limited to enzymes. Every interaction between hormone and receptor protein on the surface of an appropriate cell, every interaction between neurotransmitter and receptor protein—functioning as an ion channel—on the surface of a nerve cell, every interaction between cytokine and receptor on the surface of a sensitive cell, every interaction between foreign molecule and an immunoglobulin, every interaction between peptide and an MHC protein during T-cell recognition—all depend on this type of molecular "fit" (and in every case involves the formation of hydrogen bonds between the participating molecules to keep them in place). It is the design of molecules that are synthesized on the basis of precise knowledge about the shape of pocket or groove, and of the ability of different atoms within the amino acids that make up the pocket or groove to make hydrogen bonds with the designed molecule, that will revolutionize medical therapies in the next few decades: therapies to improve

61. Designer drugs. The figure refers to a protein that is an enzyme, neuraminidase (N). This is one of the two molecules (the other is the hemagglutinin H) found on the surface of influenza virus. The precise structure of the N protein was determined by X-ray crystallography. The left panel shows a part of the three-dimensional structure of the N protein near the active site. Bonds between individual atoms are shown as a series of straight lines. Some are brighter than others because they are nearer the surface of the molecule. Three amino acid residues—Glu 227 (glutamate at position 227 along the protein backbone of amino acids), Asp 151 (aspartate at position 151), and Glu 119 (glutamate at position 119)—are shown as thicker, tubular lines in two shades, because these are the amino acids that make contact with the molecule—neuraminic acid—that binds to N and that is altered as a result of the enzymatic action of N. The lighter shading represents carbon atoms; the darker shading represents nitrogen or oxygen atoms; hydrogen atoms are not shown. The neuraminic acid molecule, also depicted by thicker, tubular lines, is shown in the middle of the figure. Its position was determined by X-ray crystallography of a neuraminic acid–N complex. Now focus on the shaded, curved piece just below Asp 151. That is the point at which computer simulations indicate that an analogue of neuraminic acid might make contact. The molecule is 4-guanidino-Neu5Ac2en or zanamivir, and it is an inhibitor of N. The difference between zanamivir and neuraminic acid is that zanamivir has an extra group (a guanidino group) attached to it. It is this guanidino group that is predicted to bind to N. The rest of the zanamivir molecule resembles neuraminic acid so precisely that it is predicted to bind in the same places as neuraminic acid itself, and the details are not shown. The right panel shows that the predicted position of zanamivir, depicted in the left panel, is actually borne out, when X-ray crystallography of a zanamivir–N complex, shown here, is carried out. The zanamivir molecule—shown as thicker, tubular lines in two shades—sits in exactly the same position as neuraminic acid (left panel). In addition, the guanidino group of zanamivir is seen making contact with Asp 151, exactly as predicted by computer simulation. In this image only certain of the amino acids of N are shown. The figure also shows actual distances between some of the atoms of zanamivir and atoms of the neighboring amino acids of N. The distances are given in angstroms (10 angstroms = 1 nm = 1 billionth of a meter). Some of the dashed lines probably represent hydrogen bonds. Pictures courtesy of Dr. Richard Bethell of GlaxoWellcome, Medicines Research Centre, Stevenage, U.K.

---------->

61. Left.

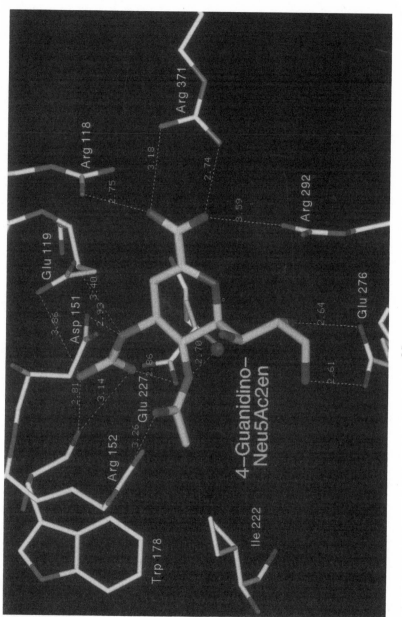

61. Right.

or dampen down molecular changes caused by disease in any tissue of the body, and therapies based on "designer vaccines" to protect against microbes that are currently still endangering life.

And what of new devices, of robotics to carry out surgery, of implants to deliver insulin or other molecule as and when the body requires it? This is a very rapidly moving field and besides presenting a few examples here, the book *21st-Century Miracle Medicine* deals with this topic in greater detail (see the Bibliography). The reader will recall mention in an earlier chapter of a monitor that measures heartbeat. Similar monitors are being produced to screen the molecules in our bloodstream and other body fluids, in order to warn of deleterious changes. Such implanted biosensors can be hooked up to a monitor so that all we need do is to watch a screen in front of us and to heed warnings like "take a sedative; you have a headache coming on," "consult your physician," or "go to a hospital *now.*" The screen could also be linked to the physician's office itself, a hospital, or the ambulance service. If all of us carry such devices in our bodies, any future involvement in a car crash could bring paramedics to the scene without anyone having to notify them.

The new techniques of genetic engineering, which are being exploited especially by biotechnology companies—the poor relations of pharmaceutical companies, since they cannot pay for huge research costs through the sale of toothpaste and deodorants—are also producing exciting results. The biggest impact over the next few years is likely to come from genetically engineered food, especially fruit and vegetables. Potatoes that contain genes designed to make us resistant to certain microbial infections, tomatoes that contain molecules to improve our sexual drive and other bodily functions—the list is endless. The problems associated with such developments are as much concerned with governmental regulations as with new technologies. Many people do not like scientists tinkering with nature—and they have a point—and are averse to eating "unnatural" foods. But is the introduction of a human gene into an apple really so different from introducing the gene of another species of apple through cross-breeding? A protein is a protein, whether produced by a piece of DNA from a human or from an apple. Most people thought it pretty unnatural when Jenner introduced cow-pox into a human being, but the technique of vaccination now saves millions of lives every year. You cannot stop the advance of knowledge, and it is difficult to stop its exploitation. There may be general agreement in terms of weapons of mass destruction, but most of us value the right of an individual to do as he wishes, provided this does not cause harm to others. Man has been inventing new technologies since he shaped the first stone tool, and has been tinkering with nature since he sowed the first field of grain. You cannot stop *Homo sapiens* from using the genes that endow us with inventiveness and drive.

In summary, the answer to the question posed earlier, is that the money spent by the pharmaceutical industry—the driving force behind designer molecules and other innovative therapies—and by governments (in other words by all of us who pay our taxes), as well as by foundations established by visionary philanthropists, is indeed producing medical advances that will improve the lives of us all. If progress seems slow, it is because the body's molecular interactions are extremely complex. Let us not forget that less than 50 years ago polio was rampant and left its victims paralyzed for life, in an iron lung or dead, that the mildest heart attack often proved fatal, and that sufferers from mental illness and stress had no recourse to any kind of drug.

———————◆———————

This chapter has considered the treatment of disease: old and new, alternative and orthodox. The message is simple: If it works for you, use it (under the care of a physician). But we cannot stand still; there is too much suffering among the diseased to ignore the molecular understanding that we are gaining daily and that opens the door to new therapies. This is the age not only of computers and the Internet, but of the possibility of improving our health in ways undreamt of a mere generation ago.

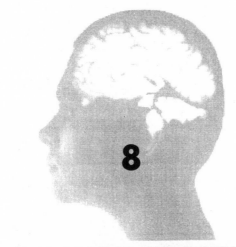

8

UNCHARTED TERRITORY

THE WORKINGS OF THE MIND

The human brain is the most highly evolved, most complicated structure in the living world. A sophisticated computer may come close to a Grand Master as far as a game of chess is concerned (Figure 62), but it will not write a novel as sweeping as Tolstoy's *War and Peace,* and it will not produce a musical score as original as Beethoven's Ninth Symphony; nor is it likely to have the intuition of an Isaac Newton or Albert Einstein. In fact, it will not produce the range of thoughts and feelings that run through our own humble brains every day: "I wonder whether Jimmy will turn out to be more like his grandfather or his uncle Bob"; "I think the reason I feel a little queasy this morning is because the tomato sauce on the pasta was too spicy last night, but then again it could be because the ice cream might have gone off a little"; "Should we go to Montana again for our summer vacation, or perhaps try Oregon for a change, or maybe go to Europe—though of course the problems with the hotel in Rome three years ago—or was it four—were pretty awful." You do not need to be a genius to have thoughts that are quite unpredictable

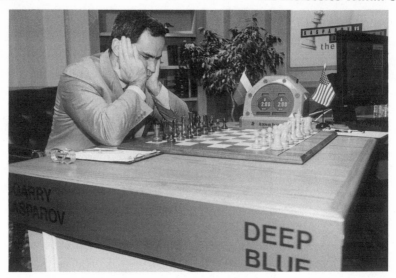

62. Human versus computer at chess. The Russian Grand Master Garry Kasparov (left) taking on the IBM supercomputer Deep Blue (right) on May 4, 1997, in New York. Kasparov had won game one the previous day. In this second game, Deep Blue defeated Kasparov after 45 moves in 3 hours and 42 minutes. It was only the second time in history that a computer program had defeated a reigning world champion. Photo by Mike Segar (Reuters).

and that encompass as wide a range of topics as those of a Thomas Jefferson or John Steinbeck. How is all of this achieved within a structure that is no bigger than a small melon?

The brain consists of almost 100 billion cells—half of which are nerve cells or neurons—all laid down during the later stages of pregnancy and within the first few years after birth. By 6 years of age the whole brain is 90% of its final size. No further neurons are produced during the rest of our life, though new connections between neurons continue to be made. On the contrary, some existing neurons start to die off as soon as we are born, during development of an intricate neuronal network. Yet what remains is sufficient to record everything we shall see, hear, feel, taste, or smell; sufficient to produce every emotion we shall experience, every thought—every dream—we shall have, every knowledge we shall acquire, over the rest of our lives. The basis of all consciousness, and of all messages that are sent from the brain to the rest of the body—messages like "move the little finger of your left hand" or "start running *now*," messages to breathe, to digest, to keep the heart going, to pass water, and so on, as well as messages from the rest of the body to the brain—the sensations of sight, sound, touch, taste, and smell—is communicated through neurons (Figure 63). What is the nature of this communication? It is nothing more than the passage of a weak electric current that passes from neuron to neuron or from neuron to cells like muscle or gland.

Biological currents—whether in a torpedo fish or a human being—are carried not by electrons, as in a metal wire or silicon chip, but by ions: ions like Na^+, K^+, Ca^{2+}, or Cl^-. We speak of ions because when a salt like sodium chloride ($NaCl$; common salt), potassium chloride (KCl), or calcium chloride ($CaCl_2$) is dissolved in water, the salt dissociates into its constituent ions. These move

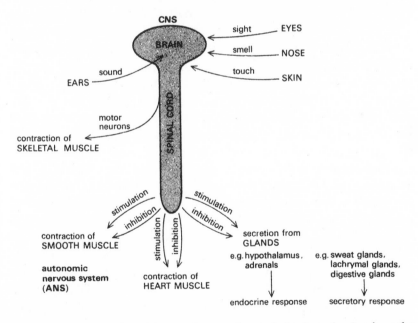

63. The nervous system. The impulses coming to the brain and going from the spinal cord to the rest of the body are indicated. From *An Introduction to Human Biochemistry* by C. A. Pasternak, Oxford University Press, 1979.

quite independently of each other, with the proviso that overall electrical neutrality is maintained, that is, the total number of positive charges is equal to the total number of negative charges. An earlier chapter referred to ion channels—made of protein—that span the plasma membrane of cells. Recall that biological membranes are made of sheets of phospholipids (Figure 13 in Chapter 2); phospholipids contain both a water-soluble or water-loving (hydrophilic) part and a fat-soluble, water-hating (hydrophobic) part. Both surfaces of the sheets make good contact with water because they contain the hydrophilic parts of phospholipid molecules; sandwiched between these two surfaces is an inner layer that is created by the hydrophobic parts of phospholipids. That inner layer creates a fatty barrier across which water and water-soluble ions and compounds do not pass. An ion channel is essentially a pore that bypasses the fatty barrier and therefore allows water and ions like Na^+, K^+, Ca^{2+}, and Cl^- to pass across the membrane. Ion channels are specific: a Na^+ channel, for example, is made up of a different protein than a K^+ channel, and so on. Moreover, there are several different types of Na^+ channels and several different types of K^+ channels, all made up of different proteins. Also, many channels consist of more than one protein— sometimes as many as five different proteins constitute a single channel. Most cells contain some of these channels, but they are particularly abundant—and important—in neurons.

A neuron is specialized in other ways. But first this discussion will summarize the ways in which a neuron is *not* specialized. In the main part of the neuron—called the cell body—there is a nucleus that contains all of the chromosomes. Outside the nucleus, within the watery cytoplasm of the cell, there are mitochondria that harness the energy produced by the oxidation of glucose—the main nutrient supply for neurons—into ATP. ATP, it will be recalled, is the universal "energy currency" of cells: The molecule provides the energy for proceses like muscle contraction, pumping ions across membranes, making proteins, RNA, and DNA, and so forth. Neurons indeed make proteins, in the manner outlined earlier: The sequence of nucleotides (A, G, C, and T) along a stretch of DNA, namely, a gene, is "read" off and translated into the sequence of amino acids that make up the protein. Although a neuron has the capacity to duplicate its DNA and to divide, it never does so; the DNA is used only to synthesize proteins as and when required. Apart from the latter point, there is nothing special about a neuron. It resembles a liver cell or a lymphocyte in the molecular changes that take place in the cell body.

Where a neuron is different is in the structure of the rest of the cell (Figure 64). It has many branches leading off it—called

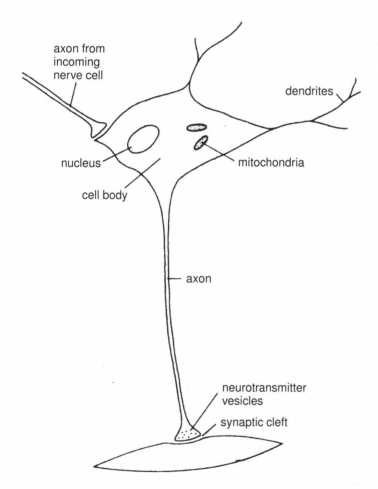

64. A neuron. From *An Introduction to Human Biochemistry* by C. A. Pasternak, Oxford University Press, 1979.

dendrites, from the Greek word for "tree"—and, in many neurons outside the brain, a larger and longer trunk called an axon. In some neurons, these are as long as a meter, which is thousands of times longer than the size of the cell body. It is through the dendrites and the axon that a neuron transmits an electrical signal or impulse to other neurons or to muscle and gland cells. The propagation of impulses depends on the function of two structures within the plasma membrane: ion channels, which have already been described here, and ion pumps.

Ion pumps are enzymes that pump ions across the plasma membrane against a concentration gradient, that is, from a weak solution to a strong one. This requires an input of energy, which is supplied by ATP; the reverse process gives off energy, and is equivalent to the loss of potential energy when an apple falls off a tree. We have met ion pumps before, in relation to the absorption of ions, water, and glucose from the kidney back into the bloodstream. One of the most important ion pumps, present in every cell of the body, is the Na^+ or sodium pump, which pumps Na^+ out of cells and at the same time pumps K^+ into cells (biochemists also refer to it as a Na^+/K^+-ATPase since it is an enzyme that uses ATP for the transport of Na^+ out of cells, simultaneously with transporting K^+ into cells). The enzyme has a binding pocket for Na^+ on the outside of the plasma membrane, and binding pockets for K^+ and for ATP on the inside of the plasma membrane, in the cytoplasm of the cell. One of the discoverers of that enzyme over 40 years ago, the Danish scientist Jens Skou (Figure 65), received the Nobel Prize for his efforts as recently as 1997. In fact, he shared the prize with two other scientists—an American, Paul Boyer (Figure 65), and a Canadian now living in Britain, John Walker (Figure 65). Boyer and Walker were studying another enzyme involving ATP. This is the enzyme that *makes* ATP, in contrast to the enzyme studied by Skou, that *uses* ATP. The enzyme that makes ATP (Figure 31 in Chapter 3) is situated in the membrane of mitochondria. It makes ATP from ADP and phosphate ions. Reactions in which ATP is degraded into ADP and phosphate ion, release energy: In the Na^+/K^+-ATPase studied by Skou, for example, that energy is used to pump Na^+ out of cells, simultaneously with pumping K^+ into cells. If degradation

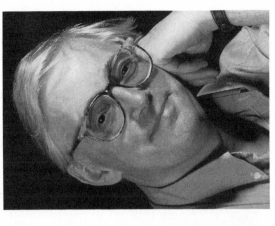

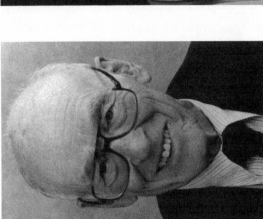

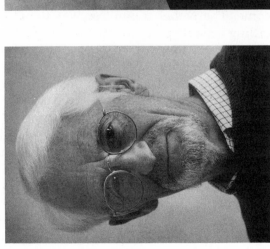

65. Jens Skou, Paul Boyer, and John Walker. Nobel laureates, 1997. Skou (left) identified the enzyme that uses ATP to pump Na$^+$ and K$^+$ across cell membranes. Boyer (center) and (right) Walker solved the mechanism by which a different enzyme makes ATP. Photographs of Boyer and Skou, copyright: The Nobel Foundation, Stockholm.

of ATP releases energy, the resynthesis of ATP must require energy. Where does it come from? The energy comes ultimately from the oxidation of foodstuffs like glucose. When glucose is being oxidized to carbon dioxide and water, the final stages of the process take place in mitochondria. During those final stages, hydrogen ions are pumped out of mitochondria into the cytoplasm of the cell. This creates an electric potential across the mitochondrial membrane that is negative on the inside, positive on the outside. The negative charge on the inside attracts H^+ back into mitochondria. They are pulled in through a special ion channel that is specific to H^+ ions. The channel forms part of the enzyme that synthesizes ATP (see Figure 31 in Chapter 3). It is the buildup of a high local concentration of H^+ that, in effect, provides the energy for the synthesis of ATP. If Skou was studying the breakdown of ATP, and Boyer and Walker were studying the synthesis of ATP, are these not two opposite, quite distinct and unrelated processes? The answer is no, they are not. The reader should understand that all chemical reactions are, in principle, reversible, irrespective of whether energy is released or required: Whether a reaction goes forwards or backwards depends solely on the concentration of the participating molecules. An enzyme—like any other catalyst—merely speeds up the rate at which the participating molecules react, be it forwards or backwards. Since an enzyme does not supply energy, it does not influence the outcome. The Nobel committee was therefore not irrational in awarding a single prize to groups studying opposing processes.

As a result of the operation of the sodium pump, the concentration of ions on the inside of cells is not the same as on the outside. Blood and other body fluids are high in Na^+ and low in K^+, whereas the inside of cells is high in K^+ and low in Na^+. This means that Na^+ will tend to leak into cells, and K^+ to leak out, each through its respective ion channel. Because the Na^+ channel is generally closed, no Na^+ leaks in; the K^+ channel, on the other hand, is often slightly open and some K^+ tends to leak out. This creates a slight deficit of positive charges on the inside of the cell compared with the outside, and an electric potential is created across the membrane: negative inside, positive outside, just like across the mitochondrial membrane mentioned above. The plasma membranes of most cells are polarized in this way, with a membrane potential of around –70 millivolts (mV) across the plasma membrane of a neuron being typical; note that because the membrane is so thin, this potential is equivalent to 100,000 volts per centimeter, or 250,000 volts per inch, a pretty formidable voltage. What further distinguishes a neuron from other cells is that it is capable of propagating an electric impulse along its dendrites and its axon. The way this happens is as follows.

A neuron is activated at its cell body or at a dendrite by a neurotransmitter released from an adjacent neuron across a narrow gap called a synapse. A synapse is typically 10–20 nm wide (approximately 1/1000th of the width of the cell body), so the molecules do not have far to travel (Figure 66). A neurotransmitter molecule binds to the protein that constitutes an ion channel; some thousands of these are clustered at the site of the synapse. Binding between neurotransmitter and its receptor protein is similar to binding between a reactant molecule and an enzyme, or between a foreign molecule and an immunoglobulin: In each case the molecules bind because of a particularly good "fit" between them. The "lock and key" analogy for this binding was the farsighted concept of German scientist Paul Ehrlich 100 years

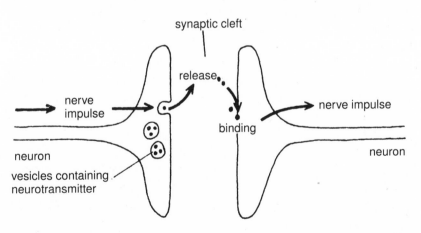

66. Mechanism of neurotransmission. From *An Introduction to Human Biochemistry* by C. A. Pasternak, Oxford University Press, 1979.

ago, and such a concept is especially appropriate in the case of neurotransmitter binding to its receptor protein because the result is literally like the opening of a door: The channel, which was previously closed, is now open. The actual movement involved is not very great: A rearrangement of some of the amino acid residues at the site of the binding is sufficient to create the difference between a closed and an open channel. Remember that it is only ions that flow through the channel, and these are not very large—about the size of a water molecule. In the case of a typical neuron that transmits signals from the brain to one of our muscles, the channels are K^+ channels. As soon as they open, K^+ ions flood out of the cell. The result of losing positively charged ions from within the neuron causes the negative charge at the inner surface of its plasma membrane to rise even higher: The membrane potential reaches around −90 mV. The difference between the previous "resting" membrane potential of −70 mV and the new one of −90 mV is somehow sensed by the proteins that comprise the Na^+ channels, and these now also open. In this case it is not so much a key that opens the door, but a bit of dynamite used by a safecracker. The result is that Na^+ ions flood into the cell and the membrane potential drops precipitously, past 0 to around +30 mV. The new potential that is set up spreads all of the way along the axon until it reaches a synapse at the other end. The plasma membrane at this part of the axon contains voltage-sensitive channels, like the Na^+ channels at the other end, except that they are Ca^{2+} channels. Because the concentration of Ca^{2+} outside cells is some 10,000 times higher than inside cells, a Ca^{2+} channel that opens up allows millions of Ca^{2+} ions to flood in. In order to appreciate the way that ions like K^+, Na^+, and Ca^{2+} flood through their respective channels from a high concentration to a low concentration, one should imagine the doors that open to be at the bottom of a dam: The pressure created by the height of water is quite analogous to the pressure created by a difference in concentration. The effect of an increase in Ca^{2+} concentration at this part of the neuron is to cause the release of neurotransmitter across the next synapse, which may be to another neuron, or to a muscle (be it heart, skeletal, or smooth muscle) or a gland cell (like the part of the adrenal that releases epinephrine). While the impulse is being propagated along the axon, the Na^+ and K^+ channels at the cell body close, and the resting membrane potential of -70 mV is reestablished within 1/1000th of a second.

The essential details of this remarkable mechanism were worked out almost half a century ago—when molecular analysis of events in cells was still in its infancy—by two English scientists, Alan Hodgkin (not the man who gave his name to Hodgkin's disease; he lived 100 years earlier) and Andrew Huxley (brother of the novelist Aldous Huxley) (Figure 67). They worked not with axons from human beings or experimental animals like cats and dogs, because the size of such axons is too small for them to have been able to insert the electrodes available at the time to measure the current passing along an axon. Instead they turned to squid, which has exceptionally large axons required to stimulate the powerful muscles that it uses to kill its prey. They reasoned that the unity of nature through evolution

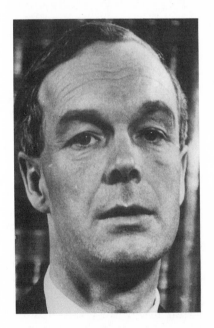
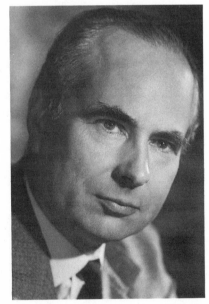

67. Alan Hodgkin and Andrew Huxley. Nobel laureates, 1963. Hodgkin is on the left. Together they identified the way nerve impulses are transmitted. Copyright: The Nobel Foundation, Stockholm.

meant that whatever mechanism they discovered in a squid was likely to be true of man also; Huxley, after all, was a descendant of the Thomas Huxley who promoted Darwin's theory of evolution in the last century. And they turned out to be right. Every impulse passed from neuron to neuron, or from neuron to muscle, in every species of animal observed to date, works through the mechanism discovered by Hodgkin and Huxley.

What of events at the terminal end of the axon? The Ca^{2+} channels close again and the extra Ca^{2+} that has leaked into the neuron is pumped out again by an ATP-driven Ca^{2+} pump. The neurotransmitter that is released—acetylcholine in the case of all skeletal muscles—across the synapse binds to its receptor in the plasma membrane of the muscle cell. That receptor is a Ca^{2+} channel, which opens up and Ca^{2+} floods in. This causes the muscle fibers to contract through an ATP-driven mechanism. A simple experiment carried out half a century ago by two Hungarian scientists, Bruno Straub and Albert Szent-Györgyi, showed that a drop of ATP added to an isolated muscle fiber lying on a glass slide caused the fiber to contract. Szent-Györgyi (Figure 68) was a versatile man who had already won a Nobel Prize, not for discovering how energy fuels the contraction of muscle, but for elucidating the molecular structure of vitamin C (ascorbic acid). Szent-Györgyi was one of the many scientists who left Germany and Eastern Europe during the period between 1930 and 1960, driven out first by Hitler and then by Stalin. Countries such as Britain and the United States, which received many talented scientists like Szent-Györgyi, in what was probably the biggest migration of intellectuals in history, have little reason to regret their generosity: Their scientific base flourished to an extent that made them the leading nations in terms of science and technology in the world. Only in the last few decades has scientific excellence been reborn in Germany and the Eastern European countries; at the same time it has blossomed in Japan.

The details of muscle contraction are quite complicated. They involve several proteins in addition to the two main constituents, namely, the proteins actin and myosin. The way that actin and myosin slide over each other during the contraction of

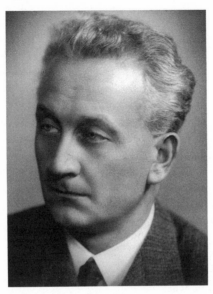

68. Albert Szent-Györgyi. Nobel laureate, 1937, for his characterization of ascorbic acid (vitamin C). Later, Bruno Straub and Szent-Györgyi showed that isolated muscle fibers contract when ATP is added to them. Copyright: The Nobel Foundation, Stockholm.

a muscle fiber is shown in Figure 69. They slide back again during the relaxation of the fiber, which happens spontaneously without an electric impulse. The details were worked out largely by Hugh Huxley (no relation), an English scientist now living in the United States (Figure 70). The whole process of conduction from brain to muscle is extremely fast. This is because the impulse generated at the cell body of an axon is not diminished as it travels along its length; the reason is that the axon, like wire in an electric cable, is well insulated: The insulating material is nothing other than layer upon layer of plasma membrane wound around the axon like a bandage. The plasma membrane—which as we have seen has excellent insulating properties because of its fatty (hydrophobic) layer in the middle—is made by cells that lie adjacent to the axon, rather like toothpaste being pushed out of its tube. Because of the insulation, an impulse can be propagated along an axon at a rate of 100 meters a second (which is over 200

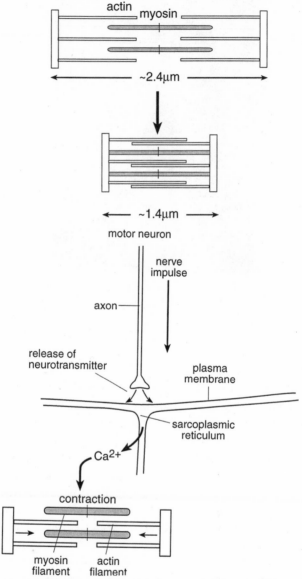

69. Mechanism of muscle contraction. The upper picture shows how filaments of the proteins actin and myosin interact by sliding past each other during muscle contraction. The lower picture shows how calcium (Ca^{2+}) triggers the process of contraction. From *An Introduction to Human Biochemistry* by C. A. Pasternak, Oxford University Press, 1979.

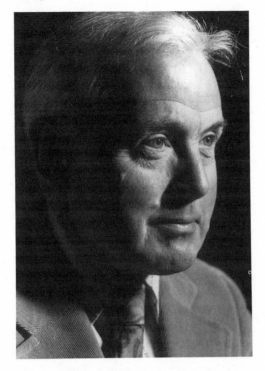

70. Hugh Huxley. Photograph lent by Dr. Huxley.

miles per hour). This means that an impulse from brain to toe can arrive in less than a tenth of a second. Without the insulating layers, called a myelin sheath, conduction is much slower; in axons that do not have a myelin sheath, impulses travel as slowly as half a meter a second. If the insulating sheath of a myelinated axon becomes damaged, the speed of conduction is reduced. This is what happens in multiple sclerosis, one of several demyelinating diseases in which areas of myelin become destroyed—often through an autoimmune mechanism as described in Chapter 5— and muscle contraction becomes irregular and slow.

The text has described in some detail how impulses emanating in our brain cause our muscles to contract for two reasons: first because the impulses travel farther than in any other situation, and second because the mechanism is typical of all forms of

nerve conduction in the body. Transmission of impulses to skeletal muscles is called voluntary: We make a conscious decision to
contract the muscles of our face—to move our eyes, to grin or
frown, to cough or sneeze, to yawn or wrinkle our nose (some
people can also move their ears); to contract the muscles of our
neck—to look over our shoulder or at our feet or into the sky; to
contract the muscles of our back—to bend or twist our body; to
contract the muscles of our limbs—to stretch our arms, to wriggle our fingers or toes, to move our legs. The reader may consider
that some of these movements are not really voluntary, since they
happen without much thought on our part. But the point is that
we *do* have control over them. We *can* suppress a sneeze, stifle a
yawn, or refrain from moving our legs. In contrast, transmission
to the muscles of the heart—to keep it beating—and to the muscles of the gut—to cause contractions that drive food from stomach through the intestines (best observed when watching a snake
that has just swallowed a rabbit)—is involuntary. Other involuntary impulses travel to organs that are in part controlled by the
brain, like kidney, bladder, lung, and spleen and to secretory
glands like the adrenal (secretion of epinephrine) and those
responsible for the secretions from our eyes (tears), nose (mucus),
and mouth (saliva).

Most of the activities just described—whether voluntary or
involuntary—depend on impulses that reach the brain from the
rest of the body: impulses of sight from the eyes, sound from the
ears, smell from the nose, and taste from the mouth, and impulses of touch and pain, heat and cold, from the skin and all
other parts of the body. Pain and heat may be closely connected.
The molecule capsaicin, which is the active ingredient of hot chili
peppers, appears to act on the same membrane receptor (causing
an influx of Ca^{2+} as well as of Na^+) as does heat. The consequence
of eating capsaicin that is perceived in the brain is the same as
that perceived by intense heat: pain. Because capsaicin acts on
the neurons that are responsible for the pain of neuralgia (like
postherpetic neuralgia that was mentioned in an earlier chapter),
and because the influx of Ca^{2+} following capsaicin may lead to
the inactivation of those neurons, "designer" molecules based on
capsaicin, which inactivate without causing too much pain, may

prove to be valuable in the treatment of neuralgia and similar ailments. All of these impulses that have been mentioned, are received and coordinated in various parts of the cerebral cortex.

The whole brain is an extremely delicate, soft—almost mushy—organ that extends into the spinal cord; parts are gray and other parts are white (a high concentration of myelinated axons gives these parts a whitish color). The spinal cord continues down the body as far as the pelvic region below the small of the back. Nerves to the muscles of the lower extremities emanate from here, so that the longest axons are those between the pelvic region and the toes. The brain and spinal cord are protected against accidental injury not just by the hard, bony structures of the skull and vertebral column or backbone, but within these casings by several layers of tissue, filled with fluid (cerebrospinal fluid), called the meninges. The meninges surround every part of brain and spinal cord, so that these delicate structures literally float, like a ship's compass, within its lining. The part of the brain that joins it to the spinal cord is known as the brainstem and is the most important in the sense that if it is badly injured, none of the rest of the brain and therefore none of the rest of the body including the heart, continues to function. Behind the brainstem is a mass of tissue known as the cerebellum. Above the brainstem, and extending somewhat around it is the major part of the brain—the cerebrum (Figure 71). The outer lining of the cerebrum, which is so convoluted that it makes up nearly half of the cerebrum, is the cerebral cortex. The incoming sensory nerves are concentrated in different parts of the cerebral cortex: visual nerves at the back, auditory nerves in the middle, taste nerves just above, and the sensory nerves from skin and the rest of the body above that.

We have seen that in any one neuron there are likely to be at least three types of ion channels: a K^+ channel, a Na^+ channel, and a Ca^{2+} channel; some neurons also have a Cl^- channel. The channels are opened either by a neurotransmitter and/or by a change in the potential across the membrane, as described above for the propagation of an impulse along an axon. The Cl^- channel is often closed, rather than opened, by neurotransmitter. Although there are different subclasses of each of these channels, with slightly different properties reflecting differences in the molecu-

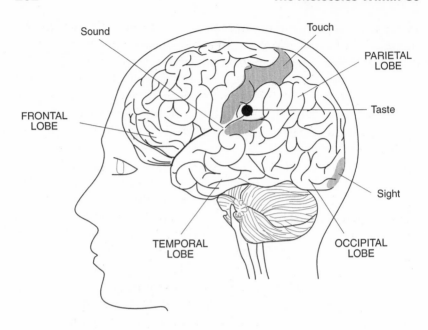

71. The human brain. The primary sensory areas of the cerebral cortex are indicated. The structure beneath the cerebral cortex is the cerebellum; it surrounds the brainstem, which leads at its lower end into the spinal cord. Adapted from *Human Physiology* (6th edition) by A. J. Vander, J. H. Sherman, and D. S. Luciano, McGraw–Hill, 1994.

lar makeup of the proteins that constitute the channels, the total number of different channels is still relatively small. Even allowing for the fact that one ion channel may have binding sites for more than one type of neurotransmitter or regulatory molecule, the whole spectrum of ion channel responses to stimulation is limited to a few dozen. In other words, if we are looking for an explanation of the vast range of stimuli and thoughts that we experience every second of our waking day, it is not in the molecular nature of the ion channels that conduct impulses.

Ion channels are not the only target of neurotransmitter action. Enzymes in the plasma membrane of the cells that are stimulated by them are another. In this instance the result is modulation of neuronal impulses, rather than initiation of an impulse. The neurotransmitter does not bind directly to the enzyme; it binds to a special receptor protein in the plasma membrane, and that receptor protein binds to another protein (called a G protein), which binds to the enzyme. It is as though you have three dominoes standing behind each other; you push the first, and eventually the third one falls over. So it is with membrane proteins. In this instance binding leads to a subtle change in shape of the respective protein, so that its interaction with the next protein is favored. The end result of all of these interactions is that an enzyme becomes activated. There are three types of enzymes. One breaks down a particular type of phospholipid that is present on the inside of the plasma membrane; the other two cause molecular rearrangements in two nucleotides that are present in the watery cytoplasm of the cell. One of the nucleotides is ATP; the rearrangement that occurs (to form a molecule of cyclic AMP) is quite unrelated to the role of ATP as an energy-transducing molecule. The other nucleotide is GTP (G instead of A); in this case GTP is broken down to form GDP and phosphate (in some cells there is also another change, leading to cyclic GMP). In all of these cases the products of the enzymatic reaction act as "second messenger" within the cell (the "first messenger" being the neurotransmitter) (Figure 72). The actions just described are not confined to neurotransmitters; they are also the most common mechanism by which hormones, like the "fear and flight" hormone epinephrine, exert their action. This should not surprise us, for we know that epinephrine acts as a hormone on liver—to stimulate glycogen degradation for extra energy— and as a neurotransmitter on neurons. The action at the plasma membrane of cells is the same in each case; what differs is the effect of the second messenger. Liver cells are preprogrammed such that an increase in second messenger activates the enzymes of glycogen degradation; neurons are preprogrammed so that an increase in second messenger affects an ion channel; the channel can be situated near the cell body where it propagates an impulse, or at the end of the axon where Ca^{2+} channels cause the release of another neurotransmitter. Of the three enzymes mentioned, each may be activated by several different neurotransmitters, but the total number of combinations is less than

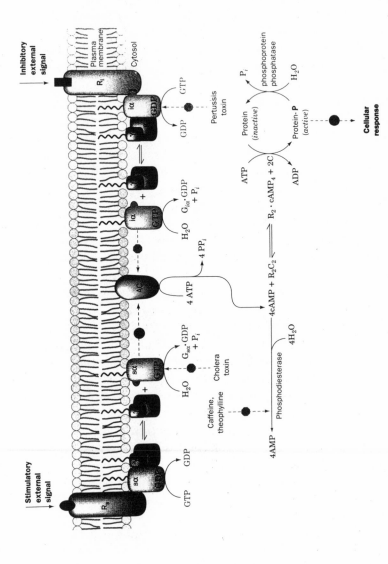

72. Cell signaling. The proteins that span the plasma membrane bind the first messenger. This results in binding of the membrane-spanning proteins to other proteins that generate the second messenger, like cyclic AMP (cAMP). This causes phosphate to be added to certain proteins that then initiate a cellular response. The action of various bacterial toxins (cholera and pertussis) and drugs (caffeine and theophylline) in modulating the cellular response is indicated. From *Biochemistry* (2nd edition) by Donald and Judith Voet, John Wiley & Sons, Inc., 1995, with permission.

100. Again, insufficient to account for the vast variety of impulses in the brain.

What of the neurotransmitters themselves? Nine different classes are known, and although there are several variants in each family, the total does not exceed 100. It is worth pausing for a moment to describe their molecular structures and the type of neural activity that they elicit. All are either amino acids or peptides, or are derivatives of an amino acid (Figure 73). This is another example of the molecular economy of nature. As animals having a nervous system started to evolve some billion years ago, the same molecules that had been the building blocks of proteins in their ancestors for several billion years were used: Consider epinephrine and the close derivative norepinephrine; both function as neurotransmitters in the brain, as well as in many neurons outside the brain. They are derived from the amino acid phenylalanine, which is a precursor of another amino acid, tyrosine.

Another neurotransmitter derived from phenylalanine or tyrosine—similar to epinephrine and norepinephrine—is dopamine. This functions in areas of the cerebrum, where neurons controlling movement and posture originate. Such a role for dopamine is compatible with its involvement in Parkinson's disease: Patients, who number approximately 1% of the population over 55, suffer from a characteristic tremor (the disease used to be known as shaking palsy), muscle rigidity, and difficulty in movement. Their problems are ameliorated by administration of dopa, which is the metabolic precursor of dopamine. It is now clear that in Parkinson's disease, there is severe degeneration of dopamine neurons—up to 90% in some areas of the brain—for reasons that are not well understood. Autoimmune destruction could be one cause. An alternative therapy for Parkinson's patients is not to supply the missing neurotransmitter, but the cells that make it. Grafting of such cells—from the brains of aborted fetuses—has been pioneered in Sweden and has led to some encouraging recoveries. The problems have been less with rejection by the immune system (the brain takes to foreign cells relatively well) than with rejection by some communities, who view the use of fetal tissue as immoral and encouraging abortion. Defective transmission by dopamine

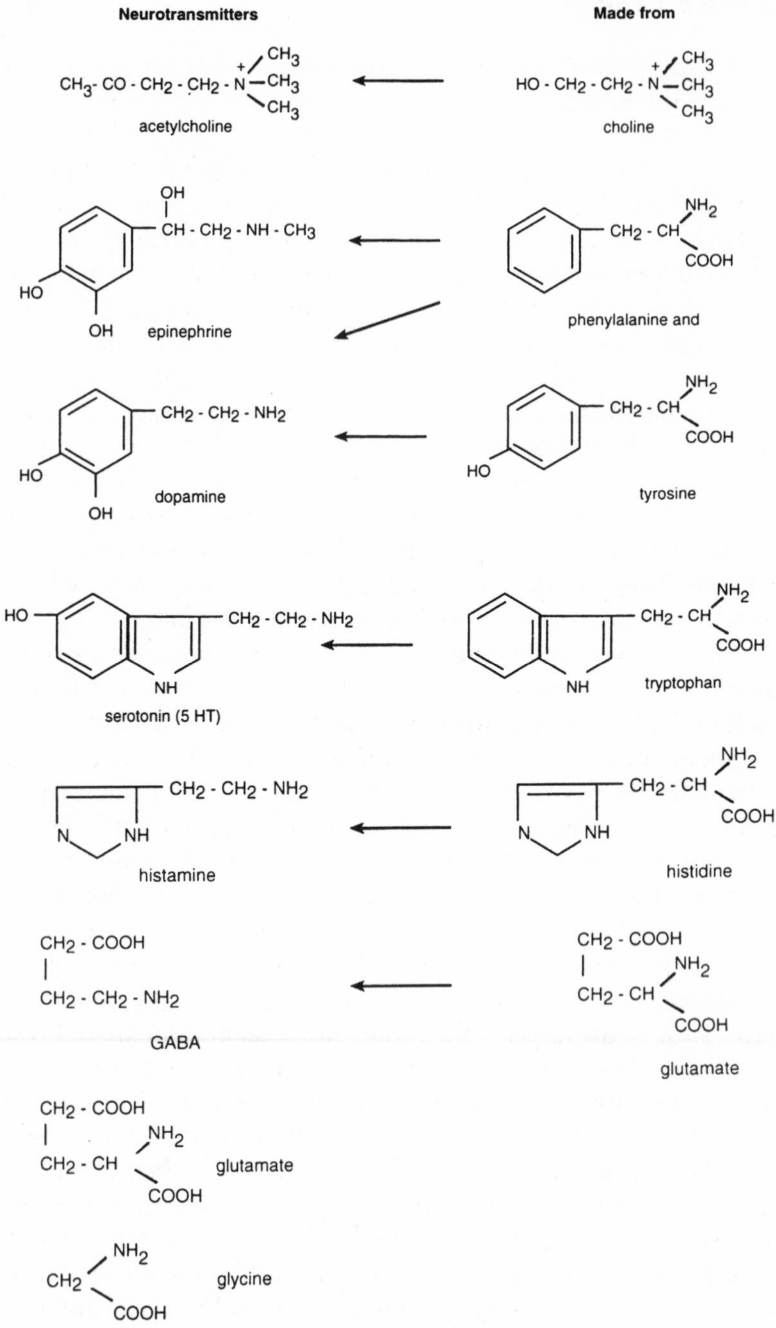

Neurotransmitters   **Made from**

$CH_3\text{-}CO\text{-}CH_2\text{-}CH_2\text{-}N^+\overset{\displaystyle CH_3}{\underset{\displaystyle CH_3}{-CH_3}}$ ⟵ $HO\text{-}CH_2\text{-}CH_2\text{-}N^+\overset{\displaystyle CH_3}{\underset{\displaystyle CH_3}{-CH_3}}$

acetylcholine   choline

epinephrine ⟵ phenylalanine and

OH
|
CH-CH$_2$-NH-CH$_3$

HO

OH   epinephrine

$CH_2\text{-}CH\overset{\displaystyle NH_2}{\underset{\displaystyle COOH}{}}$

phenylalanine and

CH$_2$-CH$_2$-NH$_2$

HO

OH   dopamine

$CH_2\text{-}CH\overset{\displaystyle NH_2}{\underset{\displaystyle COOH}{}}$

HO

tyrosine

HO— [indole ring] —CH$_2$-CH$_2$-NH$_2$

NH

serotonin (5 HT)

[indole ring] —$CH_2\text{-}CH\overset{\displaystyle NH_2}{\underset{\displaystyle COOH}{}}$

NH   tryptophan

[imidazole ring] —CH$_2$-CH$_2$-NH$_2$

N   NH

histamine

[imidazole ring] —$CH_2\text{-}CH\overset{\displaystyle NH_2}{\underset{\displaystyle COOH}{}}$

N   NH

histidine

CH$_2$-COOH
|
CH$_2$-CH$_2$-NH$_2$

GABA

CH$_2$-COOH
|
$CH_2\text{-}CH\overset{\displaystyle NH_2}{\underset{\displaystyle COOH}{}}$

glutamate

CH$_2$-COOH
|
$CH_2\text{-}CH\overset{\displaystyle NH_2}{\underset{\displaystyle COOH}{}}$ glutamate

$CH_2\overset{\displaystyle NH_2}{\underset{\displaystyle COOH}{}}$ glycine

73. Neurotransmitters.

appears to play a part also in stress-related anxiety and depression, since inhibitors of the enzyme that breaks down dopamine (monoamine oxidase)—in short that prolong the activity of dopamine by inhibiting its destruction—have proved beneficial. The opposite state of affairs—excessive dopamine transmission—may be a causative factor in the development of schizophrenia. If this proves to be the case, we will have identified a molecular target for the design of appropriate drugs.

Two amino acids, glutamate and glycine, are neurotransmitters in their own right. Both act mainly in the brain, glutamate to open channels and cause excitation of neurons, glycine to close channels and cause inhibition. These effects can take place on one and the same channel: Whether it opens or closes depends on the ratio between glutamate and glycine at their respective binding sites on the channel protein. Glutamate, which is the most abundant amino acid in brain and probably accounts for the majority of neuronal impulses, also controls neuronal activity via a second messenger system as described above (Figure 72). The affected neurons appear to be involved in neurodegenerative disorders like Huntington's disease or the secondary effects of AIDS. Huntington's disease is a particularly relentless progressive disorder, which usually starts in middle life. It is characterized by jerky movements involving the head, face, and limbs; dementia is a common feature. An amino acid derivative that is increased in AIDS is quinolinic acid, derived from tryptophan. Its concentration in the fluid inside the spine (cerebrospinal fluid) increases dramatically in AIDS patients. This is especially true for those who are suffering from an opportunistic infection, because of the failure of the immune system, or who are suffering from dementia, which is likely caused by quinolinic acid. Both dementia and secondary infections decline through treatment with AZT, a drug with some efficacy against AIDS.

An amino acid that we have met before, in connection with the action of sedative, antianxiety drugs like the diazepines, is GABA. GABA is produced from glutamate (Figure 73) and, like glutamate, is widely distributed throughout brain and the spinal cord. Its main receptor is a Cl^- channel, which it inhibits. Apart from anxiety symptoms, GABA has been implicated in Huntington's disease, Parkinson's disease, epilepsy, senile dementia, and schizophrenia.

Acetylcholine is a neurotransmitter that has wide action, like epinephrine and norepinephrine, outside the brain; the beating of the heart, for example, and all movements of skeletal muscle are triggered by acetylcholine. Although the body can synthesize acetylcholine from the amino acid glycine, most of it is derived directly from choline (Figure 73), present in foods like meat, fish, or dairy products. Acetylcholine neurons are found in the cerebral cortex and other parts of the brain; Figure 74 illustrates the distribution of those neurons in the brain. Their extensiveness shows that acetylcholine triggers many different responses in the brain. Similar "maps" of neurotransmitter action may be plotted for all of the other neurotransmitters of the brain. One of the functions of acetylcholine is in pain perception.

Serotonin (5-hydroxytryptamine), like quinolinic acid, is derived from the amino acid tryptophan (Figure 73). Unlike quinolinic acid, most of it is found outside the brain and, indeed, outside the nervous system in a number of different cell types. Its structure resembles the psychedelic drug LSD and for this and other reasons it is associated very much with patterns of elevated mood (serotonin receptors are the target for drugs like LSD). Clinical conditions resulting from an alteration in serotonin function include anxiety and other stress disorders, eating disorders, migraine, pain sensitivity, schizophrenia, sexual disorders, sleep disorders, and several other symptoms. Neurons that are triggered by serotonin are found in the cerebral cortex, cerebellum, and the regions in between. There are more than a dozen types of serotonin receptors, which function mainly through second messengers; one receptor directly affects an ion channel. In other words, serotonin controls whether the channel is open or closed.

Histamine, formed from the amino acid histidine (Figure 73), resembles serotonin in that it is distributed largely in cells outside the brain. Only relatively recently has its neuronal function in the brain been understood, through its presence in cerebral cortex and underlying areas like hippocampus (so-called after the Greek word for "sea horse," which the structure resembles), thalamus, and hypothalamus. Histamine controls neural

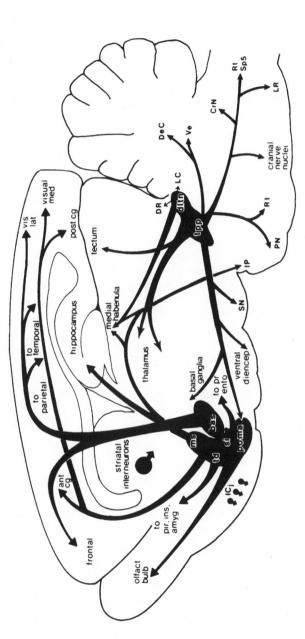

74. Acetylcholine neurons in brain. Schematic representation of the major cholinergic systems (involving neurotransmission by acetylcholine) in the brain. The extensive number of cholinergic pathways includes local and more distant circuits. Enzymes involved in synthesis and degradation of acetylcholine were stained by a variety of techniques. Adapted from L. L. Butcher and N. J. Woolf in *The Biological Substrates of Alzheimer's Disease* (A. B. Scheibel and A. F. Wechsler, eds.), pp. 73–86, Academic Press, New York, 1986 and N. J. Woolf and L. L. Butcher in *The Biological Substrates of Alzheimer's Disease* (A. B. Scheibel and A F. Wechsler, eds.) pp. 73–86, Academic Press, New York, 1989 and reproduced from *The Biochemical Basis of Neuropharmacology* (7th edition) by J. R. Cooper, F. E. Bloom, and R. H. Roth. Copyright 1970, 1974, 1978, 1982, 1986, 1991, 1996 by Oxford University Press, Inc. Used by permission of Oxford University Press, Inc.

activity through receptors that activate second messengers, and that result in the control of appetite, arousal, and other functions. This is to be expected, since antihistamines (prescribed largely for asthma and hay fever) induce hunger and drowsiness.

Peptides such as the endorphins and enkephalins, derived from precursor proteins, have already been mentioned in regard to stress. Of course it is only to be expected that molecules involved in the symptoms of stress should play a role as neurotransmitters in the brain. We have also seen that endorphins and enkephalins were identified as being the molecules, synthesized in the body, that interact with the receptors for opioids like morphine and heroin, which are situated in various sites of the brain. Those receptors function, at various sites in the brain (as well as outside, in the control of fluid movement in the gut, for example) through second messengers. Given that endorphins and enkephalins share receptors with morphine, it is not surprising that they function—among other things—in the control of pain. Indeed, one of the endorphins is 100 times more powerful an analgesic than morphine. Naturally it was hoped that knowledge of the molecular structure of enkephalins and endorphins might lead to novel drugs with which to fight addiction to morphine and heroin, but so far the results have been disappointing.

What may be learned from this discussion of neurotransmitter structure and function is much about the unity of mechanisms underlying nerve impulses in the brain. But it was diversity, not unity, that was the objective in trying to explain the myriad of different impulses coursing through our brains. The conclusion is clear: Diversity is not to be found in structural differences between the participating molecules: not in ion channel proteins, not in receptor proteins that trigger second messengers, not in the structures of the different transmitters. Where, then, can it lie? The most likely answer—and this admission itself shows that we do not yet know—is in the *pattern* of connections between different neurons, and in the *usage* of those neurons. We saw earlier that any one neuron may make many connections, through the dendritic processes that each have a synapse at their end through which impulses are transmitted to many more neurons: In the brain, some neurons receive as many as 100,000 different inputs from neighboring neurons. The complexity of such neural networks is staggering. But so are the networks of sophisticated computers, and these function not through 100 or so variables as in our brain, but on just a single mechanism: the passage of electrons along a silicon chip. So it is not unreasonable to suppose that much of the versatility of feeling and thought reflects the possibility of following one or other out of billions of different pathways. How those pathways are chosen is as yet quite unclear. And what of the usage of those pathways, since we intuitively feel that usage has somehow something to do with learning? Again, we are in mystery land, but some clues are beginning to emerge.

First it should be said that learning, and retention of what has been learned, has been tracked to parts of the cerebral cortex and particularly to the underlying region of the hippocampus. Neurotransmitters like acetylcholine, norepinephrine, and glutamate enhance long-term memory, while GABA inhibits it. Alzheimer's disease, which is present in half of the population aged over 85, is associated with a loss of memory, failure to recognize objects and people, and inability to orient oneself in time and space. Acetylcholine neurons in the hippocampus degenerate, and the protein called β-amyloid accumulates in the form of insoluble fibers within cells. Once these deposits accumulate, it is difficult to remove them, but failure of acetylcholine transmission should lend itself to a pharmaceutical approach—by administering drugs that mimic its action, or drugs that prevent its degradation, for example; sad to say, such approaches have not been successful to date. At the same time it appears that a particular cytokine (tissue growth factor or TGF-β1) is elevated in Alzheimer's and this may be directly related to β-amyloid deposits. Lowering of TGF-β1, or designing anti-TGF-β1 molecules, is therefore another approach worth pursuing.

A technique that looks promising in the area of learning and other mental functions is positron emission tomography (PET). In this technique, the emission of a type of elementary particle called a positron from certain radioactive isotopes—such as glucose containing ^{11}C in place of ^{12}C—is measured. The technique is harmless for two reasons: First, it is very sensitive, so that the radioisotope needs to be introduced in only tiny, "tracer" amounts; second, positrons are very short-lived and give rise to innocuous products, namely, photons, which forms the basis for detecting the radioisotope. Nevertheless, the technique cannot be said to be noninvasive, and for that reason was not mentioned earlier. What PET studies have shown is that when certain parts of the brain are activated, there is increased blood flow in very precise regions of the brain, indicating an increased demand for energy at these sites. Figure 75 illustrates the effect of lightly touching the fingers of one hand to their thumb. Similar results have been obtained merely by thinking certain thoughts. On the other hand, it has been calculated that the amount of extra energy actually used up by spending the entire day solving mathematical equations can be met by eating a few peanuts! Clearly the efficiency with which neurons use their source of energy is limited. PET is useful not only for tracking different mental activities to different parts of the brain and therefore localizing the participating neurons, but also for identifying which parts of the brain are used by different neurotransmitters, as described above, and which parts are involved in different diseases, like Parkinson's disease.

If learning is one part of the story, forgetting is another: A disease like Alzheimer's is an obvious example. But there are other situations that are far less distressing, but mystifying nonetheless and more difficult to explain in molecular terms. Four years ago a middle-aged man from Massachusetts was involved in a serious car crash. When he recovered, he found himself speaking with a French accent, even though he had never traveled farther than New Jersey. Other cases include British people sounding Mexican, a Norwegian sounding German, a Czech sounding Polish, a Portuguese American sounding Chinese, and, most recently, a Scotswoman speaking with a South African accent. The result of too much television watching buried in our brains, perhaps? In each case some injury like a mild stroke preceded the change. Comedians who delight us with their imitations of famous people beware: You may wake up one day unable to throw off the speech of your quarry!

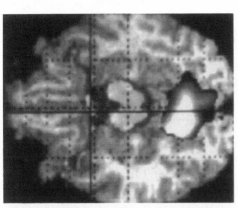

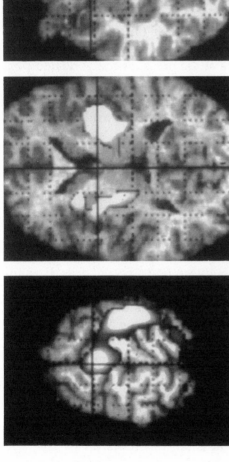

75. PET scan of brain. Three "slices" of the brain of a male volunteer were analyzed by positron emission tomography (PET) and superimposed on the same slices visualized by MRI (see Figure 58 in Chapter 7). The reduction in size is the same in all three pictures. The front of the brain is at the top of the picture and the back of the brain is at the bottom. Left picture: near the top of the brain. Middle picture: middle of brain (corresponding to a line running through the tops of the ears and the eyebrows). Right picture: a little bit above the middle picture. The subject touched each finger of his right hand to the thumb of that hand and kept doing so for about 90 seconds. During that time, saline in radioactive water [in which some of the normal oxygen (^{16}O) is replaced by radioactive oxygen (^{15}O)] was injected into his left arm to measure blood flow in different areas of the brain. The overall process was repeated six times, with rest periods in between. The pictures produced during rest were subtracted from those during movement. The white blobs indicate areas in which blood flow was increased by movement of the fingers. Left picture: extra blood flow is seen in the middle (the motor cortex) and in the lower right (sensory area). Middle picture: extra blood flow is seen in the middle on the right (basal ganglia) and in smaller areas in the middle on the left. Right picture: extra blood flow is seen in the middle of the bottom (basal ganglia in cerebellum) and smaller ones in the middle. The conclusion is that a relatively slight muscular movement—touching thumb and finger—induces increased blood flow in several areas of the brain. Picture courtesy of Drs. Sureen Rajeswaran and David Brooks, MRC Cyclotron Unit, Department of Neurology, Royal Postgraduate Medical School at the Hammersmith Hospital, London.

How does usage of particular pathways within the brain relate to possible molecular changes during learning, especially long-term memory? It is possible that the second messenger systems referred to earlier are involved. One of the consequences of triggering these systems is that some proteins become phosphorylated (i.e., get a phosphate residue attached at certain amino acids; see Figure 72). Could it be that as one learns, and uses the same neurons over and over again, some proteins become more and more phosphorylated, and that the ability to recall what one has learned is promoted by the extent to which these proteins have had phosphate residues attached? And that forgetting involves loss of phosphate residues, over time, of the same proteins? Such a mechanism of molecular "imprinting" is at least plausible, if without evidence at the present time. A related possibility is that not only does the degree of phosphorylation of a particular protein change during learning—or the concentration of some other molecule build up—but that quite different and as yet unidentified proteins become synthesized within neurons and that their presence, maintenance, or subsequent decay is associated with learning, memory, or loss of memory, respectively. Such a scenario has received some impetus recently from the identification—so far only in the fruit fly *Drosophila*—of a protein that is involved in associative memory; that is to say, in linking two stimuli—like smell and touch—together, and then remembering them. The protein is involved in cell signaling (Figure 72) and also in forming contacts between two adjacent cells. If a similar protein is found in our brain, and many of the proteins first recognized in *Drosophila* have turned out to have counterparts in the human body, it would be a good candidate for a role in learning and memory. This, of course, does not solve the problem of distinguishing one thought from another. However, we should not forget the diversity of millions of different proteins—the immunoglobulins and related proteins on lymphocytes—that are generated through fairly simple mechanisms of recombining relatively few gene products during the maturation of the immune system. In short, that there is, after all, in neurons a vast diversity of molecules—as yet undiscovered proteins—that are involved as modulators of neural activity in our brain. What tends to make this somewhat unlikely is the fact that diversity in the immune system is generated during repeated rounds of cell division, and neurons do not divide.

Perhaps we will have to settle for changes in the pattern of synaptic contacts (remember the 100,000 synaptic contacts to one neuron) after all; that is, every time a particular synapse is used, the neurons on either side of the synapse somehow "remember" the event. But what is the molecular nature of remembering, of maintaining one pattern as opposed to another? We are back at molecular imprinting, and all of our experience of molecular memory in the control of events in other cells, points to the buildup of a molecule—or the extent to which it becomes modified—to some threshold level; in other words, two events, like two thoughts, might increase the concentration of a certain molecule to a value, say of 2. If the concentration does not increase above 2, the molecule decays away. But if the concentration reaches the threshold level of 4—through two more thoughts— this might be high enough for it to bind to some other molecule, like a protein. Such an event might then trigger another molecular change through which the combination of four thoughts is remembered. Certainly we know that for a molecule to bind to a protein and initiate a reaction—be it the action of an enzyme, a hormone, an immunoglobulin, or a neurotransmitter—requires a threshold concentration of the molecule to be present; below the threshold there is no response. As yet, the simple answer is that we do not know enough about the events underlying learning and memory. And if we are still in ignorance about the molecular basis of learning and memory, we do not even *begin* to understand the processes that underlie changes of mood—depression and joy, anger and love—every emotion we experience during our waking (and sleeping) moments. We thought that knowledge of the way that drugs like LSD or morphine, Valium or Prozac, work would yield a clue, and so far that is about all they have done. They have pointed in a general way to the type of neurotransmitters that are likely to be involved, but as for more precise details, we are still waiting. If ever there is an area of biology that is ready for a breakthrough, be it a new technique or a novel concept, it is in the molecular events in our neurons that underlie thought and mood.

—————————◆————————

This chapter has been devoted to giving an overview of how nerve impulses are generated and transmitted. The molecular events that have been described account for inputs from our senses to the brain, and for outputs from the brain to our muscles and the rest of our body reasonably well. For a molecular explanation of our thoughts and emotions, the reader will have to patiently await a second—or a third—edition of this book; but if he or she is young enough to be around in 2050 (the author is not), there is little doubt that the molecular changes that elude us today will have been revealed.

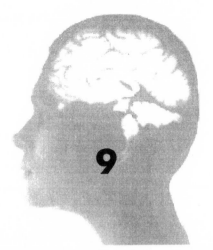

MATURATION, AGING, AND DEATH

Our body is not a fixed structure. For the first 18 years or so, from the moment an egg is fertilized by a sperm and starts to grow in the womb, through birth and into adulthood, new tissues and new organs are being laid down. But even after that, there is turnover of many tissues in that some cells are degraded and replaced by new ones. A cut on the skin is repaired, a sunburnt skin returns to normal. Inside our body repair goes on as well: The cells lining the alimentary tract are continually being sloughed off and replaced; the same is true of the cells lining all parts of the respiratory system. An infection or an inflammation leads to the recruitment of white cells to the site of injury; when the cells have completed their task, they die off and are eventually replaced by new ones. Within cells, molecules are continually being replaced. A glucose molecule has a life of minutes. A protein molecule has a life of hours, days, or months, depending on its function: Enzymes turn over fast, structural proteins like actin, myosin, or collagen, slowly. RNA is turning over fast, as new proteins are made. Only DNA remains stable, without any turnover. What changes are superimposed on this continual wear and tear of our molecules, as we mature in childhood, and as we age in adulthood? These are the questions that are addressed in this chapter.

Throughout fetal life the body grows continually: all cells are dividing and at the same time differentiating into the organs that make up the newborn: brain, lungs, heart, liver, muscles, kidneys, gastrointestinal tract, and so on. Some cells will continue to divide frequently: the precursors of the red and white blood cells in the bone marrow, the cells lining the surfaces of the gastrointestinal and respiratory tracts. Others will divide occasionally: the cells of lung, heart, liver, and kidney. Yet others will not divide at all: the cells of skeletal muscle and those of brain, spinal cord, and nerves in the rest of the body. And some cells will actually begin to die off: the cells of the brain, and the cells of the thymus.

The thymus, situated in the upper part of the chest, is, we have seen, an important organ of the immune system: It is where T lymphocytes are processed. The main reason for the destruction of cells in the thymus—which starts already in late fetal development and continues in the young newborn—is the destruction of those T cells that react to the body's own proteins. During this time all of the proteins of the blood, as well as cellular proteins and their peptide degradation products, are being presented to the T cells. In the thymus those T cells are then selectively destroyed by a mechanism that is not yet clear. At this time, the newborn is therefore particularly vulnerable to infection, which is why it is preferable to breast-feed an infant whenever possible, as the mother's milk contains immunoglobulins that are able to ward off at least some bacterial infections. It may be noted that an infant's intestine does not constitute as impenetrable a barrier to undigested proteins as later on in life. In other words, intact proteins are able to be absorbed into the bloodstream to initiate an immune response. Even in adulthood, some proteins such as oral polio vaccine are able to reach sites that initiate an immune response. This is achieved largely through the type of immunoglobulin called A, which is present in mucus secretions in the alimentary tract and in milk. Maternal immunoglobulins (of the A type) can therefore penetrate to an infant's immune system and destroy invading microbes.

The T lymphocytes that recognize our own proteins continue to be destroyed for some time and the whole thymus, as well as other lymphoid organs like the tonsils, gradually decline as puberty is reached. By adulthood, the thymus is down to 10% of its original size. Killing of T cells in this way is not a random process, but a very orderly one of programmed cell death known as *apoptosis* (a Greek word used to describe such processes as leaves falling off a tree in the fall). In this way any cells that could mount an immune attack against our body tissues and organs later on are destroyed. Apoptosis is therefore different from the uncontrolled killing of cells by microbes or toxic chemicals. Apoptosis occurs also in the cells of brain, during the growth of cancer cells (mostly they either divide and grow or die), and probably throughout later life as the aging process becomes ever more dominant. Blocking apoptosis, for example, prevents blindness (so far shown only in the fruit fly *Drosophila)* and may slow other degenerative processes associated with aging in our bodies also.

We are all familiar with the phrase "we start to age the minute we are born" and to a certain extent it is true. Not just the specialized cells of thymus and brain, but every cell within us. As already described, the longer the egg cells in the ovaries are exposed to environmental effects like background radiation, the more likely are mutations in DNA to arise. There is no reason to suppose that this gradual accumulation of damage to DNA, in effect an accumulation of mutations, is limited to the female germ cells: Every cell in the body is at risk. This statement encapsulates the "error hypothesis of aging," which proposes an accumulation of errors in DNA to underlie the aging process. Errors in the structure of DNA—an A turned into a G, or a T missing, for example—are passed via RNA to proteins. If the error occurs in a gene, a protein that functions less well may be formed; if it occurs in a control region near a gene, a hormonal stimulus may fail to switch on the synthesis of a particular protein. And if proteins are faulty, cells do not work as well as they should. The effect of DNA damage is greatest in those cells—like egg cells—that do not divide, because there is then no opportunity for the repair enzymes, which correct errors during DNA duplication, to work.

Another mechanism by which aging takes place is oxygen. This may come as a surprise, especially when recalling the emphasis in earlier chapters on oxygen as the very breath of life. Can it also be the kiss of death? The role of oxygen in aging is not as crucial as it is to life: Rather it represents a very minor, though not insignificant, side reaction. The way this comes about is as follows. The major enzymes in the body—within the mitochondria—which reduce oxygen to water during the process of turning the energy derived by the oxidation of glucose and fat to ATP, cause no damage; they are crucial to our survival. However, there are present outside the mitochondria, in the cytoplasm of cells, enzymes that reduce oxygen not all of the way to water, but only part of the way to molecules like superoxide, or rather superoxide ion (negatively charged, like chloride ion), O_2^-. These are rather unstable, short-lived molecules of high reactivity called free radicals, which combine readily with other molecules. One of those molecules is water, for the free radical combines with the first molecule it bumps into; since there are some 10,000 more water molecules in cells than any other molecule like glucose or ATP, it is with water that the free radicals will combine. The result of that reaction—it is so rapid it occurs without the need for an enzyme—is hydrogen peroxide or H_2O_2. Hydrogen peroxide is a powerful oxidizing agent: For many blondes (Marilyn Monroe used to be among them) it is hydrogen peroxide that helps them to achieve that hair color. Recent research shows the success of their efforts: Dyed blondes are said to have more fun, worry less about money, and are ruder than their counterparts with natural hair color. However, you should be aware that frequent contact with hydrogen peroxide is likely to age your skin faster, just like too much sunbathing.

Hydrogen peroxide, which is a much longer-lived molecule than free radicals, starts to damage organic molecules—again nonenzymatically—indiscriminately: molecules like DNA, proteins, phospholipids, and so forth. Where there are repair enzymes, as for DNA, damage may not be serious; nor will it be serious if the molecule has a short life, i.e., if it is constantly being degraded and resynthesized anyway. But where this is not the case, and the phospholipids of the plasma membrane seem to be particular targets, subtle changes will leave the damaged molecule less able to perform its function properly. And a less efficient cell is, in essence, an aged cell. Because of the potential danger of a free radical like superoxide arising from oxygen, our body contains an enzyme, superoxide dismutase, that destroys superoxide; whether or not damage occurs depends on the relative amount of superoxide dismutase that is present, and how quickly it can reach its target. Vitamin E and preparations containing the element selenium are also (in concentrations higher than the normal) able to mop up free radicals, so these preparations are on the "complementary medicine" counters of pharmacies and drugstores as antiaging remedies. The situation is rather reminiscent of that described for zinc in an earlier chapter. However, any time you're considering increasing the concentration of any chemical, element, or vitamin, you should consult your physician first.

There is another side to the story of free radicals, or reactive oxygen species, as they are sometimes called. It now appears that one of the consequences of activating the protein p53, is to activate an enzyme that produces reactive oxygen species. Activating p53, you will recall, is one of the aims of anticancer therapy. This is because p53 is an important molecule in the process that commits cells to stop dividing: insufficient p53, or an altered p53, and cells begin to divide indiscriminately; for that reason p53 has been regarded as a tumor (cancer) suppressor molecule. Recent research shows that reactive oxygen species damage mitochondria, making them leaky and less able to make ATP. Loss of an energy supply is an early trigger of apoptosis and cell death. So if we are able to induce free radical formation specifically in cancer cells, this becomes a beneficial, not a detrimental, situation.

This discussion has mentioned two molecular processes arising from environmental influences that age the molecules within us: accumulation of random errors in DNA and the formation of free radicals. They are not unrelated, since free radicals are one likely cause of errors, that is, mutations, in DNA. Free radicals may arise from diet, from sunlight, and from other causes. If the molecules within us do not function properly, then nor do our cells. Hence, some of our cells do not work as well at age 50 as at age 25. Is there nothing we can do about this? Recent headlines have pointed to the fact that scientists are able to make cells survive longer than they normally would. Actually we have known for several decades that certain viruses—Epstein–Barr virus, a relative of herpesvirus, is one—are able to "immortalize" cells. Such cells live forever: They have defeated the biological clock that is inside many cells, by which they undergo just so many rounds of cell division, but no more. The molecular mechanism by which this occurs is being unraveled. It appears to be related to the removal of a few nucleotides (the building blocks of DNA) from the ends of chromosomes: At every cell division chromosomes become a little shorter. Eventually the length reaches a threshold, beyond which cell division ceases. In cancer cells, this biological clock appears to be bypassed or even reversed, so cancer cells continue to divide forever. (The reader may wonder why chromosomes do not get shorter at every generation: If they did, they would have shrunk to a very small size by now, some thousands of generations having passed since man walked out of Africa. In fact, the original length is made good in our germ cells during the process of producing eggs or sperm.) So if we can prevent the biological clock from working, can we not endow our cells with longevity? Possibly. But remember two things. First, unrestricted growth is a stimulus for turning a normal cell into a cancer cell. Second, it is a pretty tall order to change every cell in our body in such a way that the coordination between liver and heart, kidney and muscle, is retained. In any case, loss of cell division is not part of the aging process. Most cells in our brain never divide anyway, yet degeneration of mental activity is a common—and one of the most debilitating—aspect of aging.

What other environmental influences affect aging? Pollution, infections and stress surely play their part. In addition there may be a mechanism in our genes that actively promotes aging processes. So far such genes have not been identified, but it is a possibility that we await with interest as the Human Genome Project proceeds to identify all of the genes within our chromosomes. If such a mechanism does exist, it will be difficult to keep the aging process at bay merely with vitamin E and selenium. Either way, we should really not be surprised that our functions gradually become less efficient with time: that some cells die off, that certain proteins do not work as well as they might, that neuronal function concerned with memory begins to deteriorate, that our immune system is not as robust at 70 as it is at 17. On the contrary, what should surprise us is the incredible durability of some of our organs, especially the heart. The muscles of the heart contract and expand, in order to drive over 5 liters of fluid around our body against a pressure of some 100 mm of mercury, 36,792,000 times in 1 year—without stopping or once missing a beat; that is over 2.5 billion times by age 70 in a healthy person. Earlier on we compared the heart to a central heating system that drives water around a house. Can you think of any circulating pump—or indeed of any other man-made machine—that is able to match this kind of performance, without ever stopping for maintenance or replacement of parts, in the remotest degree?

But some changes do take place. Gradually our arteries do begin to fill up with atheromatous deposits, no matter how healthy our diet, and the risk of heart failure does increase with age. The response of the heart to exercise—strongly recommended to maintain it in a healthy condition—declines with age because its muscles, like our skeletal muscles, no longer respond to exercise in the same way. When we are young, we are able to increase our cardiac output from the resting value of about 5 liters a minute (which means that the entire amount of blood in our system is pumped around the body every minute) to 35 liters a minute during strenuous exercise; note that the change is in the *amount* of blood pumped, not in the *rate* at which it is being pumped: The heartbeat may increase by only a few percent. The increase in output is the result of a feedback mechanism, part hormonal, part neural, that exists between the organs of the body and the heart. In exercise it is related entirely to the fact that the muscles are consuming glucose (or other nutrient like fatty acids) and oxygen at a much faster rate than at rest. While such demand on the heart is beneficial, because it strengthens the heart muscles, this is true only if one works up to this degree of exercise slowly. If not, it is positively damaging to the heart, and we are all familiar with individuals who lead a fairly sedentary lifestyle and then, at the first heavy fall of snow in winter, go out and shovel their driveway clear. The result? As often as not, a severe heart attack. As we age, the ability to increase heart output in the way described above, diminishes. But there is no doubt that moderate, regular exercise is as beneficial to the elderly as to the young. It is also clear that restricting our caloric intake—eating less—slows down the aging process and age-related diseases.

Aging affects our skeletal muscles also. Regular exercise strengthens skeletal muscles, by improving their capacity to burn up nutrients like glucose and fatty acids to make ATP; it is ATP that provides the energy for muscle contraction. That is to say, more mitochondria are made, and the muscles gradually thicken (recall the bulging muscles of weightlifters). The actual muscle fibers do not change, as there is no increased synthesis of the muscle proteins actin and myosin. As we age, the ability to enlarge our muscles decreases, and the actual force that our muscles are able to generate decreases also: by about 30 to 40% between ages 30 and 80.

In general, there is a redistribution of mass between tissues like muscle and fat as we age: Muscle mass decreases, but adipose tissue, the number of fat cells, increases. The skin becomes thinner, and wrinkles appear. Because a wrinkled face is associated with an aged face, we do not find it so attractive. There is an inbuilt mechanism within us—as in all animals—that makes us prefer youth to age for a sexual partner. We may venerate old people for their wisdom (less prevalent nowadays than it was in, say, ancient Greece: the term old fogy is more often on our lips than seer). However, men's abilty to produce sperm can last well into their 80s, producing healthy children. In general, though, men lose their sexual ability—if not their urge—around the same time as women: 2% of American men are impotent (unable to achieve an erection) at age 40; by age 65 that number has increased to 25%. (But help is at hand in the form of a drug called Viagra.) Can the menopause, which typically starts around age 50, be delayed? Male readers are reminded that the menopause causes major changes only in the ability of women to conceive: Sexual urge is not diminished and may even increase. In principle the menopause may be delayed or offset by the administration of female hormones like estrogen and similar molecules, known as hormone replacement therapy or HRT. You do not even need to take expensive pills: A couple of slices of Australian soya and linseed bread—available in bakeries of the northern hemisphere as well—contain as much estrogen as any HRT pill (surprise number one, plants contain estrogenlike molecules; surprise number two, they substitute for human estrogens). But there is a downside to this: As levels of estrogen increase, so do the chances of developing a cancer of the uterus or breasts. This is offset by a greater benefit in avoiding heart disease and osteoporosis. There is no escaping the fact that our body is delicately poised between molecular benefits to one organ and molecular damage to another. Fruit growers face a similar choice; do you go for size at the expense of taste, or color at the expense of shelf life? Better knowledge of the precise molecular features of target cells in our body will enable pharmaceutical companies to design more efficient drugs that are aimed at specific cells, with fewer side effects on other cells, in the future. Currently, then, there is much interest on the side of pharmaceutical companies to come up with a safe treatment for delaying the menopause. Career women increasingly delay starting a family until after they have made their mark in their chosen profession, and delaying the menopause would be an attractive option in certain cases. But the amount of money and effort spent on delaying the menopause pales into insignificance with that devoted to eradicating wrinkles.

Face-lifts have been around for a considerable time and have provided a healthy living for many plastic surgeons. Their monopoly or hold on the beauty industry is, however, at threat. The player that entered the stage around 15 years ago is a protein called collagen. It is a fibrous molecule that is secreted by connective tissue cells or fibroblasts; these lie just beneath the cells that line the inner surfaces of blood vessels, respiratory and gastrointestinal tracts, and are also present in muscle and every organ of the body. Connective tissue cells and the molecules like collagen (the most abundant protein in our body), which are secreted into the spaces between cells, literally form the connections between different types of cells and thereby confer rigidity and shape on the various organs within the body. During aging there is a loss of elasticity and a thinning of cartilage. This can lead to osteoarthritis, a crippling and painful disease of the joints, especially in those of the hand and hips. It can also cause calcium deposits in the cartilage of the chest wall, so that it is less easy to expand it during breathing; on the other hand, bones become more brittle. Connective tissue cells also lie beneath the cells that form the surface of skin.

The observation that by injecting collagen just below the skin, it could be stretched somewhat, like in a face-lift, and therefore improve the appearance, was a milestone in cosmetics; an entire company, devoted solely to producing collagen in the right configuration and in sterile condition, was set up in California. The disadvantage to the patient—though not quite so disadvantageous to the practitioner—is that collagen is gradually resorbed by the body, and after a year the whole process has to be repeated. In order to avoid this, preparations based on polymers containing silicon, which are not biodegradable, are gradually replacing collagen implants. These are supplemented with lipids in the form of vesicles; the preparations are made thinner or thicker depending on the site of injection, thinner for lips, thicker for nose or mouth, and so forth. The ability to remove wrinkles at specific sites at will—on the forehead, beneath the eyes, the mouth, the neck, wherever—is an obvious advance over an entire face-lift. But what is threatening the plastic surgeon—the professional—is that the techniques of collagen implantations and other cosmetic procedures can be carried out by trained paramedics in a relatively simple way, with local anesthetics to minimize pain. (Of course one needs to be very careful in determining the qualifications of such would-be plastic surgeons.)

In addition, of course, there are a host of "antiaging" creams available, some containing antioxidants like selenium and vitamin E to prevent free-radical formation, some containing retinol and other goodies of greater or lesser efficacy, that we are all able to apply on our own, to arms and legs as well as face. How effective are these remedies? It is difficult to say; if someone at 60 looks like 45, it *may* be because of the creams applied; on the other hand, it may also be a reflection of person-to-person variation—that is as true of aging as of all other body functions—and that the person would have looked younger than her age anyway.

But the plastic surgeon is fighting back. Listen to Brian Kinney, chairman of the Technology Committee of the American Society of Plastic and Reconstructive Surgeons talking about a novel digital camera and 3D software package that films patients' faces and then allows them to choose the kind of improvements they would like to have:

> The ideal situation for this kind of technology would be where people want their nose altered. A surgeon could take a picture of them, feed it into the computer, and then, through talking with them and understanding what they want, alter the shape of the nose until it is what they want. It means surgeons and patients will have a far better idea, in 3D, of what they are trying to obtain. The next step for this technology is taking the image and then projecting it over the person's face. The surgeon could then flick between the image of the desired look and compare it with progress made so far. He could use the overlay to judge when he has altered the eyelids or nose just enough. One of the main things that stops people considering plastic surgery is the fear that they don't know what they're going to look like. With virtual reality we could show them and accept the desired 3D image as a goal. I truly believe it is going to be central to plastic surgery in about 4 or 5 years' time, when systems are made available and then become affordable for surgeons. I predict that within 10 years plastic surgeons will have to practice on a virtual-reality machine before they are allowed to work on real patients, just like a pilot has to prove himself in a flight simulator.

There is no reason why the training element of such machines could not be developed for other operations as well: The medical student of the future will find himself sitting more in front of an "operating simulator" than standing over a real patient.

As we age, our memory starts to decline, especially that of recent events; this is compatible with the view that an "imprinting" mechanism—repeated usage of certain neural connections—is involved in memory and that it is this mechanism that begins to decline with age. Part of the trouble is that older people, when not employed, receive less intellectual stimulation. There is also a gradual slowing and loss of all higher intellectual functions. The answer as far as our intellect is concerned is simple: Use it or lose it. As might be anticipated, of course, there is a large person-to-person variation. Some people start to slow up at age 50, others are still as bright as a button at age 100. What is becoming clear is that the more we use our brain, the less likely our neurons are to degenerate. In that regard, neuronal connections are like muscles: If we don't use them, they tend to atrophy. This is itself remarkable. Can you think of a machine or an automobile, once it is run in, that improves its performance through usage, and that declines if switched off or left inside the garage (the battery of a car is an obvious exception) ? In the case of our mind, conscious exercise through tasks like playing with computers, making things with our hands, reading or writing—why do you think I am writing this book?—as opposed to staring at a television screen most of the day, will delay the aging process considerably.

We also become more susceptible to disease as we age. Our immune system is less able to protect against infecting microbes, some of our neurons begin to degenerate and leave us with a higher chance of developing Parkinson's or Alzheimer's disease, our arteries are in greater danger of precipitating a heart attack, our muscles and joints do not recover as well after a fall and do not react as rapidly to nerve impulses sent from the brain, our eyesight begins to fail because the ciliary muscles that control the shape of the lens begin to degenerate. There is no part of our body that is not affected, and very few diseases that do not become more prevalent with age. Some diseases are rarely seen in the young at all. These include osteoarthritis and osteoporosis, a condition in which bones become brittle and likely to fracture if one suffers a fall. It is most common in women following menopause and is responsible for over a million and a half fractures per year in this group in the United States alone. The reason is because the beneficial effects of estrogen on bone structure are lost. Currently there are no very effective therapies against either osteoarthritis or osteoporosis: The precise molecular defects are not yet clear, which makes the rational design of drugs difficult.

Finally, try as we may to keep our bodies fit and healthy, the reaper eventually arrives to end our brief sojourn on this planet. If we inquire into what actually causes death, failure of the heart resulting from cardiovascular disease is seen as the leading cause (Table 9). There is considerable regional variation, related predominantly to dietary differences: Among the developed countries, Finland has one of the highest rates (probably related to a high incidence of alcoholism brought on by those long winter nights) and Japan has one of the lowest (a healthy diet low in fat). Heart disease is followed by cancer, respiratory disease, accidents, and so forth. In the United States, Alzheimer's disease is moving into third place as the most common cause of death. In the less developed countries, where serious infectious diseases are still rampant because of malnutrition and poor hygiene, the rank order will be somewhat different, but heart failure will still be the most common cause of death. As already mentioned, our heart serves us incredibly well for most of our lives, but eventually it just gives up. Without the oxygen and nutrients that the heart pumps into every tissue of the body, we cannot function. The brain, as we saw at the beginning of this book, is particularly vulnerable, but a person can be virtually "brain dead" yet, provided his heart keeps going, he is still technically alive. Only when the brainstem—which controls so much of our physiology including the heart—ceases to function is the person technically (at least in some countries) dead.

Is the answer to longevity then the heart? In the sense that we can limit atheromatous deposits in our arteries, which are the

Table 9. Causes of Death in Developed Countries

Cause	Frequency
Cardiovascular disease	45%
Cancer	18%
Respiratory disease	6%
Accidents	6%
All others	25%

major cause of heart disease, through diet and a careful lifestyle, yes. In the sense that we should consider swapping our heart for a younger one if a suitable donor can be found (pigs make excellent donors, as their heart is just about the same size as ours), no. First of all, major surgery, followed by all of the attendant immunological problems, makes this a difficult procedure at the end of one's life: The body at age 80 or 90 is simply not able to cope. Second, for much the same reason, even if we obtain a healthy heart at such a ripe age, all of the other changes that accompany aging will have manifested themselves. What is the point of a new heart if we are crippled with arthritis, suffering from mental deterioration, and unable to enjoy the things we used to do at 25, 50, or even 75? The more ambitious of us will say that if we attend to each of these problems as they arise—by novel drugs, manipulation of our genes (a gene that appears to promote aging—at least in mice—has recently been identified), and treatments we cannot yet envisage—we shall be able to extend life indefinitely. This is entering into a dream world that is as unrealistic as taking the genes of a cat—why not a sunflower while we're at it—and turning them into a human being. What we shall undoubtedly see—it is happening already—is a prolongation of life by keeping disease at bay.

In 1952, 255 people celebrated their 100th birthday in Britain, and were sent a congratulatory telegram by the Queen. In 1978 the number had risen to 1772, and by 1996 the number was 4688. This means that longevity is steadily increasing twofold every 12 years (Figure 76). Is this going to be an indefinite process? Probably not. First, the curve for those reaching 100 appears to be flattening out at around 4000–5000 people per year (the values from which the figure was drawn are somewhat less than telegrams sent by the Queen; this is because they have been normalized to a constant birth rate, which has fallen slightly over the years). Second, the number of those reaching age 105 or more, is much less: only 111 (6% of those reaching 100) managed it in 1978, and even in 1996 the number was only 530 (11% of those reaching 100). Why did longevity take off so rapidly after 1946? Before that date, the number of people reaching 100 was almost static (Figure 76). Partly this is the result of better medical treatment for the elderly.

Remember that Britain introduced its National Health Service at about this time. But it is unlikely to be the sole cause. A clue to what another cause might be emerges if one looks at the wages (adjusted for inflation and purchasing power) of Britons in the last century. The figures from around 1770 onwards are fairly accurate, and they show a slow increase in wages of about 20% between 1770 and 1845. Thereafter the increase jumps more than sixfold, to around 1.7% per year for at least the next 35 years; the reforms being enacted in Britain in the middle of the last century had a major and sustained effect on the real wealth—or lack of poverty—of its population. In other words, a dramatic increase in wages from 1845 onwards exactly matches a dramatic increase in those living to be 100 from 1946 onwards. One does not need to be a mathematical genius to realize that those reaching age 100 in 1946 were born in 1846. How does the increased prosperity of a mother giving birth to a baby affect that baby's chance to reach 100? The chances are that pregnant mothers ate better after 1845, and as a consequence the fetus inside them fared better; once the infant was born, its nutrition improved also. And recall that much

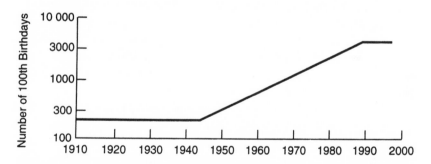

76. Increase in number of centenarians. The number of people in the United Kingdom reaching 100 was plotted against the year in which they celebrated their 100th birthday. The figures were taken from the number of congratulatory telegrams sent out by the Queen (from 1952 onwards) and from data in the Registrar General's Reports of Births, Deaths and Marriages in the United Kingdom between 1910 and 1990. The two sets of figures are in good agreement, and all lie on one line as shown. Note the break in the line at 1946 and a flattening out after 1990. Redrawn from a paper by M. F. Perutz in *Philosophical Transactions of the Royal Society of London, Series B,* **352,** 1919, 1997.

of what happens to us in later life—our stature, our mental capacity, perhaps the activity of our heart as well—depends on what happened to us in the womb and in infancy.

There is also likely to be a genetic element. First, because everyone knows that longevity tends to run in families. Second, because a team of scientists at the Gifu International Institute of Biotechnology in Japan have identified a gene that appears to correlate with longevity. The gene is carried by most Japanese centenarians, but by less than half of the rest of the Japanese population. What does the gene do? The fact that it is located, not on one of our 23 chromosomes, but on the chromosome inside our mitochondria gives a clue. For the function of the genes in mitochondria is related to supplying the energy inherent in the oxidation of sugar and fat to the rest of the cell: to enable the heart to beat through the contraction of its muscles, to enable ions to be pumped across membranes in kidney, brain, and other tissues, to enable the muscles of our limbs to contract, and so forth. In short, just as a combination of our genes and the environment contributes to the diseases that beset us, so a combination of genes and the environment contributes to health and longevity. I have analyzed in some detail the increase in longevity in Britain, simply because the figures are available. Similar trends of an increase in longevity are seen in the United States and other affluent countries; elsewhere, there is quite a bit of catching up to do. Overall, though, it is extremely unlikely that even by the end of the next century people will be living to 150 years of age as a matter of routine.

What happens to the molecules in our body when we die? Science has rejected, along with Wöhler 100 years ago, the idea that there is some vital force that distinguishes the molecules of living matter from those of nonliving matter. Do not the enzymes within our cells therefore continue to catalyze molecular reactions, even if they do not include oxidation of energy stores like glycogen and triglyceride because the supply of oxygen has ceased? That is quite correct, and while our bodies are still warm, many enzymes—especially those that degrade proteins as part of the wear and tear machinery within our cells—continue to work. Indeed, provided our bodies are not deep-frozen, many enzymes continue to work even after body temperature has fallen and rigor mortis set in. This is why we hang game out for a day or so to soften the tissues before cooking it; if left longer, bacteria and other microbes (some that were present as part of the microbial flora in the intestines of us all) take over and rancid products accumulate. Proteins are not resynthesized because there is no ATP to drive energy-requiring reactions like the synthesis of protein, nucleic acids, carbohydrate, or fat. Our bodies start to cool because the maintenance of body temperature during life depends entirely on heat liberated during energy-yielding reactions like the oxidation of foodstuffs: Only some 30% of the available energy is used for the synthesis of ATP; the other 70% keeps us warm.

As the temperature within the body approaches that of the surroundings, the reactions catalyzed by enzymes become slower and slower. If our bodies are frozen, the reactions virtually stop. This is why we freeze food (the cells of plants as well as those of animals contain degradative enzymes) and why we freeze human eggs and sperm for storage prior to *in vitro* fertilization procedures; it is also why we chill organs to be used for transplants (freezing whole organs causes irreparable damage to some of the cells). DNA, which is rather resistant to degradative enzymes, remains intact if frozen. That is why one is able to obtain samples of DNA for analysis of long-dead humans or animals once they have become buried in the permafrost of the Artic region or in the snows of sufficiently high mountains like the Alps. DNA that was originally in the precursor cells of red and white blood cells in the bone marrow survives degradation even at higher temperatures, and samples of bone recovered from peat bogs, caves, and other sites have yielded material that is still intact enough for analysis of its DNA. Eventually, however, even DNA starts to deteriorate and it is unlikely that intact specimens older than around 10,000 years will be found. The idea of obtaining, and somehow reviving, the DNA of dinosaurs that died out 65 million years ago is therefore pure fiction. But it makes a nice story, and the story makes an even nicer amount of money.

Once our bodies have cooled, the fate of the molecules within us depends on what happens to our bodies. If we die at sea, most of the flesh will eventually be eaten by fish, leaving only the skeleton behind; if one is unfortunate enough to fall into piranha-infested waters, these tiny fish—but with very sharp teeth—will devour our limbs to the bone in a matter of minutes. If we are buried on land, worms and microbes will eventually enter our coffin and—like fish—devour all organic matter. If we are cremated, the organic matter is oxidized to carbon dioxide and water; nitrogen and sulfur are oxidized to their respective oxides. The rest of the body—the skeleton, which is largely calcium phosphate, and the salts within the body fluids, which are largely sodium, potassium, and chloride—remains behind as ash. If, therefore, the reader accepts the arguments put forward in this book—that there is nothing within us except molecules—we have reached the end of our story.

Many readers will be dissatisfied at this abrupt ending and will accuse the author of writing an irreligious text (even though its substance is not too far from some of the current thinking within the Anglican Church—of which the Episcopalian Church in the United States is the closest relative). In the sense that it avoids all concepts of an afterlife, or reincarnation in some other form, this is true: If our every feeling of happiness or grief results from molecular interactions between neuronal cells, then all thought and feeling ceases when those cells are reduced to ash. On the other hand, the author has accepted religion—even if only in the mind—as a useful and satisfying experience. But it does mean that we leave nothing behind when we die. Or do we? For those of us fortunate enough to have offspring, we pass on one complete copy of our genome: 23 molecules (one of each of our chromosomes) of DNA. That in itself is somehow satisfying and counters the feeling that our presence on Earth for a limited number of years will have been a bit of a waste of time. But there is more. Whether childless or passing on our genes, we all contribute to the quality of life of those around us, and generally it is beneficial. During the writing of this book, there occurred two deaths—within a week of each other—that gripped the minds of people throughout the globe.

One was that of Diana, Princess of Wales, the other that of Mother Theresa of Calcutta; Diana was 36, Theresa 87. The world mourned both. Why? Not because it prayed for the future of their souls, nor because it prayed for the well-being of Diana's sons (though we all felt sorry for them as we would for any child bereft of its mother at an early age). The world mourned these two women because each had, in her own way, enriched our lives. But we do not need to be a well-known personality to do so. Our every action—by what we say or write or do—can give pleasure to those around us; or perturb others, as even Diana and Mother Theresa did. Still others leave a legacy of suffering and hatred, as men of evil have done through the ages. To enrich the lives of those around us—not only family and friends but also people unknown to us by name—forms a major part of all religions of the world: to give not only one's time, but also a share of one's income. By enriching the lives of others we enrich our own. In that way we may even be able to come to terms with the fear that grips us as we approach the end of our lives: What will happen to us when we die? Lucky are they who do believe in an afterlife, and who approach death with happy anticipation, not with apprehension or fear. For the rest of us, we may thank the God within us for having given us an opportunity to lead a life that has—if nothing else—been rewarding and sometimes even interesting.

This chapter has described some of the molecular changes that underlie aging and death. It cannot close with a more appropriate quotation than one written over 300 years ago by an English poet:

> Like to the falling of a star;
> Or as the flights of eagles are;
> Or like the fresh spring's gaudy hue;
> Or silver drops of morning dew;
> Or like a wind that chafes the flood;
> Or bubbles which on water stood;
> Even such is man, whose borrowed light
> Is straight called in, and paid to night.
> *The wind blows out; the bubble dies;*
> *The spring entombed in autumn lies;*
> *The dew dries up; the star is shot;*
> *The flight is past; and man forgot.*
> (Henry King, 1592–1669)

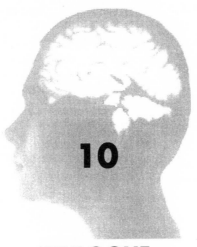

10

EPILOGUE

My aim in writing this book has been twofold: to give the reader a better picture of what goes on in his body and to enable him to plan future strategy in regard to his health. (I also owe the reader an apology. For I have shied clear of the cumbersome "he/she," "mankind/womankind," or "humankind," "they" when it is the singular that is intended, and have used words like "he" or "man" where these words could not be avoided except by interrupting the flow of the narrative. The intention throughout has been to refer to male and female on equal terms. Indeed, did I not say in Chapter 3—despite the opening of the Book of Genesis—that man appears to be made in the form of woman, not the other way around?)

The reason for choosing to describe our bodies in terms of molecules is clear. It is in molecular terms that physicians discuss many of our problems: "you should try to lower your *cholesterol*"; "your blood *glucose* is very high, so we shall have to test your *insulin* levels"; "I recommend that you take extra *iron, folic acid,* and *vitamin B_{12}* whenever your periods are particularly heavy"; "I am afraid your baby may be suffering from a deficiency of *lactase,* but the other digestive *enzymes* seem normal"; "did you realize that you have very low *factor VIII?*" It is in molecular terms that the constituents of food and medicines are described: "each slice contains 2.9 g *protein,* 10.7 g *carbohydrate* of which *sugars* are 1.1 g and *starch* 9.5 g, 0.8 g *fat* of which 0.1 g is *saturated . . .*"; "each tablet contains 200 mg *ibuprofen*"; "one tablet supplies 50,000 USP units of *amylase,* 50,000 USP units of *protease* (*trypsin* and *chymotrypsin*), and 8500 USP units of *lipase.*"

And it is in molecular terms that the most exciting medical advances are announced: "*enkephalins* mimic action of *opioid* drugs like *morphine*"; "accumulation of *β-amyloid* associated with Alzheimer's disease"; "*phosphoamides* offer new hope for cancer patients"; "novel anti*prothrombin* drug to prevent blood clots"; "*gene* for obesity related to *protein* called *leptin.*"

Knowing what different molecules associated with our body are is not sufficient. In order to understand how our body works, we need to know what these molecules do. It is the way that molecules interact with each other that underlies every function of our tissues and organs. Consider the digestion of food—predominantly carbohydrate, fat, and protein—in the alimentary tract; the absorption of digested food molecules into the bloodstream; the metabolism of those molecules to provide the energy that our body needs. That energy is required to enable our heart to beat, our muscles to contract, our kidneys to excrete unwanted products but to retain water and nutrients, our brain to think and to respond to sight, sound, touch, and smell. Energy is also required to remake carbohydrate, fat, and protein (as well as some DNA and RNA) so that the tissues of our body can be maintained, grow, and be repaired as necessary.

A healthy body is but half the picture. None of us escapes some form of illness during our lifetime. It can be as trivial as a cut or a bruise, a cold or a stomach upset, a sleepless night or a headache. But it can also be asthma or diabetes, pneumonia or malaria, a heart attack or cancer. Knowing what molecular changes are responsible for these conditions is of more than passing interest. It allows physicians to take appropriate measures in a logical manner. Equally important, it allows *us* to do the same: to decide when it is appropriate to seek treatment, and when to try to cure ourselves for some of the minor ailments mentioned above. What molecular alterations, then, underlie disease? I have emphasized the fact that very few disorders have a single cause. Most are the result of a combination of genetic or hereditary factors on the one hand, and of environmental factors such as diet, microbial infections, and stress on the other. This should not surprise us. For the way that our bodies are made in the first place is likewise dependent on a mixture of hereditary and environmental influences: whether we are tall or short, fat or thin, ambitious or lazy, clever or stupid, susceptible to certain infections or resistant to them.

The molecule responsible for inherited characteristics is DNA: Our genes are nothing more than long stretches of DNA. But DNA itself does not make our bones long or short, the tissue under our skin replete or low in fat, the neurons in our brain to function one way or the other, our immune system to recognize some microbial molecules but not others. It is the proteins within our body that do this, and the types of proteins that we make is specified by the composition of our DNA. The way this is done depends on a code, which may be compared to the Morse code (about to go out of circulation) or to the musical code. Different musical notations—a C, a D, an E flat, an F sharp, and so on— and the sequence in which they are written, code for an entire symphony, a violin concerto, or an opera. In the same way different residues in DNA—and there are just four of them, namely, A (adenine), C (cytosine), G (guanine), and T (thymine)—and the sequence in which they occur, code for proteins with complicated and diverse functions: carrying oxygen around our body (hemoglobin), controlling glucose uptake (insulin), forming muscle fibers (actin and myosin), and causing a myriad of different chemical reactions to take place (enzymes).

It is the large variety of reactions involving enzymes and other proteins that are responsible for the differences in form and function that each of us displays: reactions that cause bones to grow, fat to be deposited or burned up, hairs to be colored blond or dark, nerve impulses to be transmitted from one part of the brain or another, immune defense molecules to be made well or badly. In each case our genes specify the type and amount of protein that is made; the environment—what food we eat and how much, what microbes invade our body—dictates how well those proteins work. If we eat too much fat or insufficient vitamins, the enzymes concerned with energy production do not work properly; if we become infected with microbes, other constraints are placed on the ability of enzymes to function normally.

When we fall ill, the interplay between the genes we inherit from our parents and the environment in which we live is again played out in terms of molecules. A faulty gene, leading to the synthesis of an aberrant protein, may make us more susceptible to heart disease, to cancer, to infection, to an allergy. The molecular event that actually triggers each illness generally starts with the environment; a surfeit of dietary cholesterol or mental stress; a buildup of coal tar from cigarettes or other pollutant; a toxin produced by a streptococcus in our lungs or a malarial parasite in our red cells; an adverse molecule in our food, in the air we breathe, or on the plants we touch. To understand the molecular nature of the defect is the first stepin its prevention, treatment, or cure.

Throughout this book I have stressed the remarkable similarity in the molecular makeup of animals, plants, and microbes. While this provides the most forceful argument yet advanced in favor of Darwin's theory of evolution, and a valid reason for using animals rather than human prisoners to carry out the initial tests on the safety of new drugs and vaccines, that was not my aim. Nor was it to induce a sense of humility in ourselves in relation to our fellow creatures (though the moral superiority of *Homo sapiens* over chimpanzees or even swans—who remain faithful to each other, once they have found a mate, for the rest of their lives—is quite questionable). Rather it was to reassure the reader that introducing a molecule derived from a microbe, a plant, or another animal is as normal as boosting or depressing a molecule made in our own body. After all, we have been eating plants and animals since time immemorial, and if we can safely bypass the barrier between the alimentary tract and the bloodstream, we can deliver therapeutic molecules to where they are needed much more effectively.

My second aim has been to give the reader a flavor of some of the wonderful new diagnostics that have recently been developed, and that are likely to be refined over the next decade. Diagnosis of the molecules within our body by MRS (magnetic resonance spectroscopy); following the flow of water and other molecules through our brain and other organs by PET (positron emission tomography); monitoring molecules in our body through biosensors and relaying the information directly onto a screen in our living room; and, of course, analyzing our genes and the proteins made by them, which may predispose us to asthma or arthritis, cancer or coronary heart disease, food poisoning or flu, sepsis or stress.

And what of new therapies? Designer drugs against the ailments just mentioned; designer vaccines against HIV and hepatitis, against *Candida* and cancer, against meningitis and malaria. Some of these are already in clinical trials; others are still around the corner.

I hope I have given the reader enough information to understand the human body in molecular terms. For those who wish to delve more deeply, a bibliography of specialist books follows this chapter. If I have done no more than to remove some of the mystique of medicine—"doctor knows best: do not concern yourself with questioning our judgment"—that closes off a number of potential diagnoses and treatments, if I have done no more than whet the appetite of the reader for more information, I shall have achieved my aim. But remember this: Detailed knowledge is not everything. It is more difficult to be wise than learned, yet it is the wise person, not the learned one, who gets the most of life. As the English poet Alfred Lord Tennyson (1809–1892) put it: "Knowledge comes, but wisdom lingers."

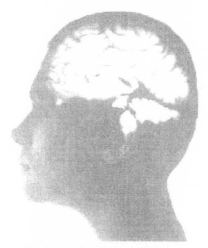

BIBLIOGRAPHY

The author has found the following books useful and recommends them to readers wishing to dig deeper into a particular subject.

B. Alberts, D. Bray, J. Lewis, M. Raff, K. Roberts, and J. D. Watson: *The Molecular Biology of the Cell* (3rd edition). Garland Publishing, 1994.

B. Alberts, D. Bray, A. Johnson, L. Lewis, M. Raff, K. Roberts, and P. Walter: *Essential Cell Biology: An Introduction to the Molecular Biology of the Cell.* Garland Publishing, 1998.

John S. Axford (editor): *Medicine.* Blackwell Science Ltd., 1996.

J. R. Cooper, F. E. Bloom, and R. H. Roth: *The Biochemical Basis of Neuropharmacology* (7th edition). Oxford University Press, 1996.

J. G. Hardman, L. E. Limbird, P. B. Molinoff, and R. W. Ruddon (editors): *Goodman and Gilman's The Pharmacological Basis of Therapeutics* (9th edition). McGraw–Hill, 1996.

S. J. Higgins, A. J. Turner, and E. J. Wood: *Biochemistry for the Medical Sciences.* Longman Group, 1994.

Brian Inglis: *A History of Medicine.* Weidenfeld and Nicolson, 1965.

Bertram G. Katzung (editor): *Basic and Clinical Pharmacology*. Prentice–Hall International, 1995.

C. Mims, J. H. L. Playfair, I. M. Roitt, D. Wakelin, and R. Williams: *Medical Microbiology*. Mosby–Year Book Europe, 1993.

Oxford Paperback Reference: *Concise Medical Dictionary* (4th edition). Oxford University Press, 1994.

John Playfair: *Infection and Immunity*. Oxford University Press, 1995.

Roy Porter (editor): *Cambridge Illustrated History of Medicine*. Cambridge University Press, 1996.

Roy J. Shephard: *Physical Activity, Training and the Immune Response*. Cooper Publishing Group, 1997.

Lubert Stryer: *Biochemistry* (4th edition). W. H. Freeman, 1995.

A. J. Vander, J. H. Sherman, and D. S. Luciano: *Human Physiology* (6th edition). McGraw–Hill, 1994.

D. J. Weatherall, J. G. G. Ledingham, and D. A. Warrell (editors): *Oxford Textbook of Medicine* (3rd edition). Oxford University Press, 1996.

Alexandra Wyke: *21st-Century Miracle Medicine*. Plenum Trade, 1997.

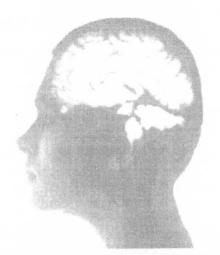

GLOSSARY OF MEDICAL AND SCIENTIFIC TERMS

The glossary found in *Biochemistry for the Medical Sciences* by S. J. Higgins, A. J. Turner, and E. J. Wood (Longman, 1994) is so appropriate to this discussion that many definitions are taken verbatim from that work, with permission. Words that are cross-referenced appear in bold.

Acetylcholine   molecule containing **choline**; a **neurotransmitter**.

Acidosis   abnormally high acidity of body tissues and fluids.

Acute   disease of rapid onset with severe symptoms and brief duration (contrast with **chronic**).

Addison's disease   weakness, loss of energy, and low blood pressure, caused by impaired secretion of **steroid** hormones by **adrenal**.

Adipose   relating to fat, e.g., adipose cells.

Adrenal   endocrine gland situated above each kidney; the adrenal cortex secretes **steroid** hormones, the adrenal medulla secretes **epinephrine** and **norepinephrine**.

Agonist   substance that triggers a response in a cell, such as a **hormone** or **neurotransmitter** (opposite, **antagonist**).

AIDS   acquired immune deficiency syndrome; disease characterized by failure to mount an immune defense against infectious microbes, that is caused by infection with **HIV** some years earlier.

Allele   one of a number of alternate forms of a **gene**.

Allergen   substance, like pollen, poison ivy, or gluten, that sets up an **immune** response in hypersensitive people, leading to **histamine** release from **mast cells** and culminating in **anaphylactic shock**.

Alzheimer's disease   neurological disorder characterized by progressive loss of short-term memory, deterioration in behavior and intellectual performance, and slowness of thought.

Amino acids   molecules that are the building blocks of **proteins**, which are made up from 20 different amino acids.

Amytal   one of the **barbiturate** group of drugs.

Anabolism   building up; making more complex molecules by biosynthesis (opposite, **catabolism**).

Anaphylactic shock   an extreme and generalized **allergic** reaction in which widespread release of **histamine** causes swelling, **edema**, constriction of the bronchioles in the lung, heart failure, circulatory collapse, and sometimes death.

Angiogenesis   formation of new blood vessels. Essential for development of a **tumor**.

Androgen   steroid **hormone** (e.g., testosterone) that stimulates the development of the male sex characteristics.

Anemia   reduction in the amount of **hemoglobin** in the blood.

Angiogram X-ray picture produced following the injection of an X-ray opaque dye into an artery.

Anoxia conditions where body tissues receive inadequate amounts of oxygen.

Antagonist inhibitor of **hormone** or **neurotransmitter** action (opposite, **agonist**).

Antibiotic a compound, usually produced by microbes, that selectively inhibits or kills other microbes (e.g., penicillin).

Antibody protein, also called **immunoglobulin**, which binds to an **antigen**.

Antigen foreign substance, like a protozoan, bacterium, or virus, which binds to an **antibody** and thereby elicits an **immune** response.

Apolipoprotein protein part of a **lipoprotein** that transports lipids in the blood.

Arteriole small artery.

Arthritis inflammation of one or more joints; includes rheumatoid arthritis (often related to **autoimmune** disease) and osteoarthritis (often related to aging).

Asthma narrowing of the airways in the lungs, leading to coughing, wheezing, and difficulty in breathing. Often brought on by an **allergen**.

Asymptomatic not showing any signs of disease, whether disease is present or not.

Ataxia unsteady gait resulting from brain's failure to regulate posture and limb movements.

Atheroma formation of fatty plaque in artery walls, which limits blood flow and predisposes to thrombosis. Atherosclerosis is a disease in which atheromatous plaques develop.

ATP adenosine triphosphate; the "energy currency" of cells, produced by the **oxidation** of foodstuffs (**glucose** and **fatty acids**) and used for muscle contraction (including the pumping of the heart), pumping of ions across membranes, and biosynthesis of molecules like **carbohydrates, triglycerides, phospholipids, proteins, RNA**, and **DNA**.

Atrophy   wasting away of a tissue or organ.

Autoimmune   disease caused by attack of certain organs or tissues by the body's own **immune** system.

Autopsy   dissection and examination of a body after death (e.g., to discover cause of death).

Autosome   any chromosome that is not a **sex chromosome** (i.e., chromosomes 1–22).

Barbiturate   group of drugs with sedative action.

Benzodiazepine   group of drugs (including **Valium** and **Librium**) that act as tranquilizers and hypnotics.

Bile   fluid from liver, stored in gallbladder and secreted into the duodenum to aid digestion of fats; contains **cholesterol** and bile acids, which are derived from cholesterol.

Bilirubin   yellow compound derived from **heme** breakdown (see **jaundice**).

Bioassay   determination of the biological activity of a compound such as a **hormone, neurotransmitter**, or drug.

Biopsy   removal of a small piece of tissue from a patient for analysis (usually carried out with a hollow needle).

Blood–brain barrier   prevents movement of many components of blood into brain and cerebrospinal fluid, and vice versa.

BSE   bovine spongiform encephalopathy, a degenerative neurological disorder of cattle, associated with an abnormal **prion** protein.

Calcification   deposition of calcium salts (e.g., in the formation of bone).

Cancer   any **malignant** tumor, like **carcinoma** or sarcoma (arising from **connective tissue**).

Capillary   narrowest type of blood vessel.

Carbohydrate   molecule made up of sugars, like **glucose**; may be a single sugar like glucose, two sugars like **lactose** or **sucrose**, or many sugars (a **polymer**) like **glycogen**.

Carcinogen   substance that produces **cancer** (see **precarcinogen**).

Carcinoma   cancer or **tumor** arising from **epithelial** cells.

Cardiovascular   system of heart plus blood vessels (pulmonary and systemic).

Catabolism   breaking down of food or storage molecules (e.g., for energy; opposite, **anabolism**).

Cataract   opacity of the lens in the eye, causing blurred vision.

Cell cycle   in dividing cells, the sequence of events between one cell division and the next.

Cerebellum   largest part of hindbrain, responsible for muscle tone and for controlling involuntary muscles.

Cerebral cortex   the intricately folded outer layer of the **cerebrum**; the cortex makes up some 40% of the brain (15 billion **neurons**) and is the part of the brain most directly responsible for consciousness, with essential roles in perception, memory, thought, mental ability, and intellect, as well for initiating voluntary activity.

Cerebrum   largest part of brain, the outer layer of which is the **cerebral cortex** (gray matter); below this is mainly white matter.

Chemotherapy   treatment of disease with chemicals; contrast **radiotherapy**.

Cholesterol   molecule present in fatty food, as well as being made in the body; see **steroid**.

Choline   molecule that is a constituent of some **phospholipids**; also a constituent of **acetylcholine**.

Chromatid   one half of a **chromosome**; a chromatid is one continuous stretch of **DNA**.

Chromosome   structure in which most of the **DNA** within a cell is packaged; there are 23 pairs of chromosomes in the majority of cells.

Chronic   disease of long duration involving slow changes, often of gradual onset (opposite, **acute**).

Cirrhosis   damage to liver, e.g., by alcohol.

CJD   Creutzfeldt–Jakob disease; a degenerative neurological disorder associated with an abnormal **prion** protein; one variant of the disease is said to be caused by eating **BSE**-infected meat.

Collagen   structural **protein** secreted by **fibroblasts**.

Coma   state of unrousable unconsciousness; the patient is said to be comatose.

Congenital   a condition present since birth.

Connective tissue   supports, binds, or separates more specialized tissues and organs; contains **fibroblasts**, fibers of **collagen** and **polymers** made up of complex **carbohydrates**; includes structures like bone and cartilage, as well as **adipose** and other types of cells.

Cornea   the transparent circular part of the front of the eyeball.

Corpuscle   a blood cell.

Cortisol   a **steroid** hormone made in the **adrenals**.

Cysteine   a sulfur (S)-containing **amino acid** that makes S–S bonds in **proteins**.

Cystic fibrosis   hereditary disease in which thick mucus obstructs pancreas and lungs; severe respiratory infections often result.

Cytokine   **protein** that acts as growth factor or other controlling molecule on cells, e.g., interferon, interleukins.

Cytosol watery interior of cells.

Dementia chronic or persistent disorder of mental function (e.g., in Alzheimer's disease).

Dermatology study and treatment of skin diseases.

Detoxification process by which toxic molecules are rendered "safe."

Diabetes mellitus disorder in which **glucose** uptake and metabolism by cells is impaired; caused by lack of, or insensitivity to, **insulin**.

Diagnosis determining a patient's disorder by signs and symptoms, medical history, tests, etc.

Differentiation increasing specialization of cells during development.

Dissemination wide distribution of pathological changes in an organ.

Distal situated away from a point of reference (opposite, **proximal**).

Diurnal occurring every day; diurnal rhythm, changes with a cycle of 24 hours.

DNA deoxyribonucleic acid; molecule made up of linear chains of **nucleotides**; **genes** are made of DNA.

Domain structurally or functionally defined part of a **protein**.

Dominant refers to an **allele** on a **chromosome** that determines the condition or **phenotype**, irrespective of the allele on the other chromosome (contrast **recessive**).

Dopamine molecule that is a **neurotransmitter**.

Down's syndrome mental subnormality, resulting from three (instead of two) copies of chromosome 21; formerly called mongolism.

Edema accumulation of fluid in body tissues; formerly called dropsy.

Effector molecule or process that brings about activity in a muscle or organ, e.g., hormone or nerve impulse.

-emia pertaining to the blood.

Encephalitis inflammation of the brain.

Endemic occurring regularly in a particular region or population.

Endocrine hormonal.

Endocytosis uptake of material into cells (opposite, **exocytosis**); also **phagocytosis.**

Endogenous originating within the body or a cell (opposite, **exogenous**).

Endorphin class of molecules, made up of many **amino acids,** i.e., a small **protein,** that act as **neurotransmitters.**

Endothelial surface lining of blood vessels and other fluid-filled cavities.

Endotoxin bacterial toxin that remains within a bacterium (contrast **exotoxin**).

Enkephalin class of molecules, made up of several **amino acids,** i.e., a **peptide,** that act as **neurotransmitters.**

Enterotoxin bacterial toxin that affects the intestine.

Enzyme protein with catalytic function.

Epidemiology study of epidemics; occurrence or spread of diseases within populations.

Epilepsy disorder of brain function producing seizures.

Epinephrine hormone secreted by **adrenal** gland, also called adrenaline.

Epithelium sheet of cells lining a surface like skin (epidermis) or alimentary tract (mucus membrane).

Erythema abnormal flushing of the skin caused by dilation of the capillaries.

Erythrocyte mature red blood cell (**corpuscle**); see also **reticulocyte**.

Erythropoiesis formation of **erythrocytes** (occurs in the bone marrow).

Esophagus tube between throat and stomach.

Etiology cause of a disease.

Exocytosis secretion of molecules from cells (opposite, **endocytosis**).

Exogenous originating outside the body or a cell (opposite, **endogenous**).

Exotoxin toxin secreted by a bacterium (opposite, **endotoxin**).

Familial condition found in some families but not others (often inherited).

Fatty acid molecule made up of a chain of carbon atoms (typically 16, 18, 20, 22, or 24 C atoms); can be saturated (all carbon atoms fully hydrogenated or reduced) or unsaturated (some carbon atoms not fully hydrogenated but partially oxidized).

Fibroblast widely distributed cell type characteristic of **connective tissue**, that secretes **collagen**.

Fibrosis thickening and scarring of **connective tissue** caused by inflammation or injury.

Fructose molecule very similar to **glucose**; a constituent of common sugar or **sucrose**.

GABA γ-aminobutyric acid, a molecule that is a **neurotransmitter**.

Galactose molecule very similar to **glucose**; constituent of **lactose**.

Gastric (gastro-) pertaining to stomach.

-gen (-genic) "giving rise to."

Gene stretch of **DNA** specifying a particular **protein**.

Genome genetic complement of an organism (including microbes); also refers to total **DNA** in an organism.

Genotype genetic constitution of an organism (see **phenotype**).

Gestation development from fertilized egg to newborn.

Glucogenic making **glucose**; e.g., some **amino acids** (contrast **ketogenic**).

Glucose molecule containing $C_6H_{12}O_6$. Most common sugar in the body; building block for **glycogen**.

Glucosuria **glucose** in the urine.

Glutamic acid an **amino acid** that is also a **neurotransmitter**.

Glutathione molecule made up of three **amino acids**, i.e., a **peptide**.

Glycerol molecule containing three carbon atoms; a constituent of **triglyceride** and **phospholipids**.

Glycine an amino acid that is also a **neurotransmitter**.

Glycogen molecule made up of many **glucose** units in highly branched form; form in which **carbohydrate** is stored in the body.

Gonadotropin a pituitary **hormone** acting on gonads (i.e., testis or ovary).

Gout painful disease associated with crystals of uric acid in tissues and joints.

Hemagglutinin substance that causes clumping together of red blood cells.

Hematology study of blood and its formation.

Heme the iron-containing molecule that is attached to the **protein** globin in **hemoglobin**.

Hemodialysis technique for removing toxic waste products from blood, usually for patients with kidney disease.

Hemoglobin the main **protein** constituent of red blood cells, that binds oxygen and carries it from the lungs to all tissues in the body.

Hemoglobinopathy disease resulting from abnormal or insufficient **hemoglobin** (see **sickle-cell disease; thalassemia**).

Hemolysis destruction of red blood cells.

Hemostasis arrest of bleeding (e.g., through coagulation).

Hepatic of the liver.

Hepatitis inflammation of the liver.

Hepatocyte main type of cell in liver.

Hepatoma **malignant** tumor of the liver.

Herpes a type of virus.

Heterozygous having inherited different **alleles** of any one **gene** from each parent (contrast **homozygous**).

Histamine molecule released from **mast cells** as part of the allergic response; causes contraction of smooth muscle, especially in the lungs, leading to **anaphylactic shock**; also has other pharmacological actions, e.g., in motion sickness.

Histology study of the structure of tissues, e.g., by staining and by microscopy.

HIV human immune deficiency virus, that leads to the onset of **AIDS**.

HLA complex human leukocyte antigen; **proteins** on the surface of cells involved in recognition of foreign compounds. If two persons have the same HLA types, they can accept each other's grafts.

Homeostasis maintenance of stable internal environment.

Homozygous having inherited the same **allele** of any one **gene** from each parent (contrast **heterozygous**).

Hormone   molecule, generally a **protein, amino acid** derivative, or **steroid**, that is secreted by one type of tissue or organ and that affects the function of another tissue or organ.

Huntington's disease   hereditary neurological disorder characterized by jerky involuntary movements, accompanied by behavioral changes and progressive **dementia**.

Hydrophilic   "water-loving"; making hydrogen bonds with water (contrast **hydrophobic**).

Hydrophobic   "water-hating," therefore "fat-loving" or **lipophilic**, making bonds with fats (contrast **hydrophilic**).

Hyper-   "raised."

Hypercholesterolemia   raised blood **cholesterol**.

Hyperglycemia   raised blood sugar (**glucose**).

Hypertension   raised blood pressure.

Hypo-   "lowered."

Hypoglycemia   lowered blood sugar (**glucose**).

Hypothyroid   subnormal activity of **thyroid**.

Hypoxia   deficiency of oxygen in tissues.

Immune   response of B and T **lymphocytes** to a foreign body like an infectious microbe, and of **mast cells** to an **allergen**.

Immunity   protection against infectious disease.

Immunoglobulin   **protein** which binds to an **antigen** or **allergen**.

Inborn error   inherited defect, e.g., of metabolism.

Infarct   death of part or all of an organ; caused by blockage of blood supply through a clot.

Inositol   molecule that is a constituent of some **phospholipids**; derivatives of inositol play a role as "second messengers," which act as signals between events at the surface of cells and subsequent events within cells.

Insulin **protein** secreted from the pancreas that promotes uptake of **glucose** into tissues.

Intravenous into a vein.

In vitro "in glass;" i.e., in a test tube, outside the body.

In vivo "in life;" i.e., inside the body.

Ion an atom that has gained a negative charge (i.e., an electron), like Cl^- (chloride), or an atom that has lost one or more negative charges, like H^+ (hydrogen ion), Na^+ (sodium ion), K^+ (potassium ion), or Ca^{2+} (calcium ion); when salts like NaCl (sodium chloride or common salt) are dissolved in water, they form a mixture of Na^+ and Cl^- ions.

Ischemia inadequate blood flow to part of the body, caused by constriction or blockage.

Jaundice yellow coloration of skin, caused by excess **bilirubin** in blood.

Ketogenic making **ketone bodies**; e.g., some **amino acids** (contrast **glucogenic**).

Ketone bodies four-carbon atom-containing compounds derived from breakdown of **fatty acids** and certain **amino acids**.

Ketosis poisoning caused by accumulation of **ketone bodies**.

Lactose molecule made up of one **glucose** and one **galactose** residue; the sugar in milk.

Laparotomy surgical incision into the abdominal cavity.

Lesion region of damaged tissue with impaired function; also used for impairment of a metabolic pathway.

Leukemia **malignant** disease in which the bone marrow produces excess immature or abnormal **leukocytes**. May be **acute** or **chronic**. Overproduction suppresses the formation of other blood cells, leading to infection, bleeding, and **anemia**.

Leukocyte white blood cell or **corpuscle**.

Librium   one of the **benzodiazepine** group of drugs.

Ligand   molecule that binds to another molecule, e.g., hormone, **neurotransmitter**, or **cytokine** binding to a receptor **protein**.

Lipophilic   "fat-loving"; similar to **hydrophobic** (contrast **hydrophilic**).

Lipoprotein   **protein**–lipid complex circulating in the blood in the form of vesicles.

Luminal   one of the **barbiturate** group of drugs.

Lymph   fluid similar to blood that bathes all tissues; main cells in lymph are **lymphocytes**.

Lymphocyte   class of **leukocyte** involved in **immunity**; the cells, called B and T according to function, are also present in lymph nodes, **spleen**, and **thymus**.

Lymphoid   tissue responsible for production of **lymphocytes**, such as lymph glands, **spleen**, and **thymus**.

Macro-   "large."

Malignant   a **tumor** that spreads and invades other tissues (contrast *benign*).

MAO inhibitors   monoamine oxidase inhibitors; group of antidepressant drugs that boost the action of monoamines like **epinephrine** and **serotonin**.

Marplan   one of the **MAO inhibitor** group of drugs.

Mast cell   cell found throughout the body in **connective tissue**; releases **histamine** and other molecules in response to inflammation or an **allergen**.

Menopause   cessation of menstruation (contrast *menarche*, the start of menstruation).

Metastasis   spread of a **malignant** tumor from its site of origin (**primary** tumor) via blood or **lymph**, often to form a **secondary** tumor.

MHC major histocompatibility complex: same as **HLA complex.**

Micro- "small."

Monoclonal immunoglobulins derived from a single **lymphocyte**, after several rounds of cell division, that are therefore identical (contrast **polyclonal**).

Monocyte a type of **leukocyte** that carries out **phagocytosis.**

Monogenic condition, often a disorder, controlled by a single **gene** (contrast **polygenic**).

Mononucleosis abnormally high number of **monocytes** in blood, as in infectious mononucleosis, commonly referred to as *glandular fever*; caused by Epstein–Barr virus.

Morbidity state of being diseased.

Morphology form and structure of the body and its organs.

Mortality (rate) incidence of death in a population in a given period.

Mutagen agent (molecule, radiation) causing a **mutation.**

Mutation change in **DNA** which may result in an altered **phenotype**; changes in germ cells are inherited, changes in other cells (**somatic** cells) are not.

Myocardium middle of the three layers that form the wall of the heart, forming the greater part of heart muscle. A myocardial infarct is a nonfunctioning segment of heart muscle following interruption of the blood supply to it (see **ischemia**).

Myxedema coarse skin, intolerance to cold, weight gain, and mental dullness resulting from underactive **thyroid** (symptoms opposite to those of **thyrotoxicosis**).

Necrosis death of some or all of the cells of an organ or tissue.

Nembutal one of the **barbiturate** group of drugs.

Neonatal newborn, within the first 4 weeks of life.

Nephron   tubule in the kidney through which filtered blood (i.e., without cells or proteins) is passed eventually to the bladder as urine; during passage through the nephron most of the water, ions, and nutrients are reabsorbed into the bloodstream.

Neuron   nerve cell.

Neurotoxic   poisonous to nerve cells (**neurons**).

Neurotransmitter   molecule involved in the transmission of nerve impulses.

Nitrogen balance   state of the body when intake of nitrogen (largely as **protein** in food) equals excretion (largely as **urea** in urine); can also be positive (when intake exceeds excretion, as during growth) or negative (when excretion exceeds intake, as during starvation).

Nodule   small swelling.

Norepinephrine   hormone secreted by **adrenal**; also acts as **neurotransmitter** in brain and elsewhere.

Nucleotide   molecules that form the building blocks of nucleic acids (**RNA** is made up of nucleotides containing ribose; **DNA** is made up of nucleotides containing deoxyribose).

Obesity   condition where excess fat, especially **subcutaneous** fat, has accumulated in the body; associated with being grossly overweight.

Olfaction   process of smelling.

Oligonucleotide   short sequence of **nucleotides**, i.e., short stretch of **DNA** or **RNA**.

Oligosaccharide   short sequence of sugars, i.e., small **carbohydrate**.

Oncogene   **gene** associated with progression toward **cancer**; oncogenes are mutated forms of normal genes.

Oncogenesis   development of an abnormal growth or **tumor**, that can be benign or **malignant**.

Osteoblast   cell that forms bone.

Osteoclast   cell that destroys or remodels bone.

Osteoporosis   loss of bone mineral resulting in brittle bones.

Oxidize   to add oxygen, or remove hydrogen, from molecules.

Palpate   examine the body by careful feeling with hands and fingertips.

Parkinson's disease   neurological disorder characterized by tremor, rigidity, and lack of spontaneous movements.

Pathogenesis   origin of a disease; a pathogen is an agent, e.g., a microbe, causing disease.

Pathology   study of disease processes by sampling and analyzing body fluids and tissues by **biopsy** and **autopsy**.

Pedigree   ancestry of a group of related individuals.

Peptide   molecule made up of several **amino acids** (typically 3–12 amino acid residues), i.e., part of a **protein**.

Peripheral   near the surface or extremities.

Peritonitis   inflammation of the membrane surrounding the abdominal cavity (that contains liver, kidneys, pancreas, and the gastrointestinal tract), often caused by a bacterial infection.

Pernicious   likely to result in death if not treated, e.g., pernicious **anemia** caused by deficiency of vitamin B_{12} related to lack of proper absorption.

Pertussis   whooping cough, caused by bacterial infection.

Phagocytosis   ingestion of material by certain **leukocytes** through the process of **endocytosis**.

Phenotype   visible or otherwise measurable characteristics of a person resulting from his or her **genotype**.

Phenylketonuria   hereditary disease (**inborn error** of metabolism) in which phenyl ketones are present in urine; characterized by mental deficiency.

Phospholipid   molecule containing two **fatty acids, glycerol,** phosphate, and a residue like **choline** or **inositol**; the fatty acids make the molecule **hydrophobic,** the rest of the molecule makes it **hydrophilic.** Together with **proteins,** phospholipids are the main components of biological membranes, such as the plasma membrane that surrounds all cells.

Plasma   straw-colored fluid in which the blood cells are suspended.

Polyclonal   immunoglobulins derived from more than one **lymphocyte,** after several rounds of cell division, that are therefore a mixture (contrast **monoclonal**); the immune response to a foreign molecule is generally polyclonal.

Polygenic   condition, often a disorder, controlled by several different **genes** (contrast **monogenic**).

Polymer   large molecule made up of many smaller building blocks, e.g., **glycogen, proteins, DNA,** and **RNA.**

Polymorph   a type of **leukocyte,** involved in **phagocytosis.**

Polymorphism   genetic character that occurs in several different forms, reflecting different **alleles.**

Porphyria   rare hereditary disorder in which **heme** breakdown is faulty.

Portal   the part of the circulation that drains blood from the intestine and delivers digested food to the liver.

Postmortem   "after death" (see **autopsy**).

Precarcinogen   substance that is converted in the body to an active **carcinogen.**

Prenatal   "before birth"; diagnosis to detect potential disease, generally inherited, by amniocentesis, chorionic villus sampling, and other techniques.

Primary   initial cause of a disease; site of original **tumor** before **metastasis** (contrast **secondary**).

Prion "infectious protein"; a **protein** molecule found normally in the body, **mutant** forms of which are associated with diseases like **BSE** in cattle and **CJD** in humans.

Protein molecule that is made up of linear chains of **amino acids**.

Proteinuria **protein** in the urine, resulting from faulty filtration of blood by kidney.

Proximal situated close to a point of reference (opposite, **distal**).

Prozac one of the **selective serotonin reuptake inhibitor** group of drugs.

Pulmonary relating to the lungs.

Radiography examination of the body using X rays and other techniques.

Radiotherapy treatment of disease with radiation; contrast **chemotherapy**.

Recessive refers to an **allele** on a **chromosome** that does not determine the condition or **phenotype**; instead this is determined by the allele on the other chromosome (contrast **dominant**).

Recombinant a form of **protein** produced by genetic engineering, e.g., human **insulin** or factor VIII produced in microbes.

Reduce to add hydrogen, or remove oxygen, from molecules.

Renal refers to the kidneys.

Reticulocyte immature precursor of red cells (**erythrocytes**).

Rickets disease of bones caused by lack of vitamin D.

Rigor mortis stiffening of the body that occurs about 8 hours after death, the result of changes in muscle tissue; starts to disappear after about 24 hours.

RNA ribonucleic acid; molecule made up of linear chains of **nucleotides**.

Rubella German measles, caused by a viral infection.

Schizophrenia severe mental disorder involving delusion and hallucinations.

Seconal one of the **barbiturate** group of drugs.

Secondary dependent or following on from another (**primary**) event; secondary tumors arise by **metastasis**.

Selective serotonin reuptake inhibitors group of antidepressant drugs that prolong the action of **serotonin**.

Sensory information carried by the nervous system to the brain.

Serotonin 5-hydroxytryptamine (5-HT), a molecule that is a **neurotransmitter**.

Serum **plasma** from which the **proteins** of the clotting system (like fibrin) have been removed by allowing the blood to clot.

Sex chromosome the X and Y chromosomes of an individual: females XX, males XY (contrast **autosome**).

Sickle-cell disease **hemoglobinopathy** in which the red cells tend to assume a sickled shape, caused by an abnormal **hemoglobin**; leads to **anemia** and **hemolysis**.

Somatic change, generally in **DNA** and therefore a **mutation**, in cells other than the germ cells (testis and ovary); not passed on to offspring.

Spleen organ situated on left side of the body, below stomach, consisting of **lymphoid** tissue and a meshwork containing red blood cells; organ in which aged red blood cells are broken down by **phagocytosis**.

Steroid molecule like **cholesterol**, or a derivative of cholesterol like **bile** acid or cortisol, that contains a characteristic ring-like structure.

Striatum region of the brain involved in the initiation of movement.

Subcutaneous   beneath the skin, e.g., subcutaneous fat.

Sucrose   molecule made up of one residue of **glucose** and one residue of **fructose**; commonly known as sugar, as in sugarcane and sugar beet.

Synapse   gap between two nerve cells, into which **neurotransmitters** are released.

Syndrome   group of symptoms characteristic of a particular disease.

Tetanus   disorder of muscle undergoing continuous contractions leading to paralysis; often caused by a bacterial toxin.

Thalassemia   type of inherited **anemia** in which **hemoglobin** production is faulty as a result of one of several defects (see **hemoglobinopathy**).

Thrombolysis   dissolution of a blood clot (thrombus) by **enzymes**.

Thymus   organ situated in upper part of body, above heart; main site where maturation of T **lymphocytes** occurs.

Thyroid   endocrine gland situated at the base of the neck secreting thyroid **hormones** (T3 and T4).

Thyrotoxicosis   increased heartbeat, sweating, tremor, anxiety, increased appetite, loss of weight, and intolerance to heat, caused by overactive **thyroid** (symptoms opposite to those of **myxedema**).

Topology   surface features.

Transformation   genetic modification of a cell leading to the formation of a **tumor**, e.g., by viruses or **carcinogens**.

Translocation   movement to another place, e.g., a piece of one **chromosome** onto another, leading to genetic disorders.

Tricyclic   group of drugs that combat anxiety symptoms; also have anti-**histamine** action.

Triglyceride   molecule made up of **glycerol** and three **fatty acids**; the main constituent of fatty foods, and of **adipose** cells.

Tumor   swelling, usually as a result of abnormal cell proliferation as in **cancer**; see **oncogenesis**.

Tumorigenesis   formation of a **tumor**.

Ultrastructure   the detailed structure of cells at the electron microscope level.

Urea   molecule derived from the breakdown of **amino acids**; the form in which most of the nitrogen in the body is excreted.

-uria   pertaining to urine.

Vaccination   process of giving a **vaccine** to immunize against an infectious disease.

Vaccine   preparation of a microbe, or a molecule derived therefrom, that leads to immunity from the disease caused by the microbe.

Valium   one of the **benzodiazepine** group of drugs.

Vasodilation   increasing the diameter of blood vessels like arteries, which leads to lowering of blood pressure (opposite, *vasoconstriction*).

Venule   small vein.

Xenobiotic   substance that is foreign to the human body; applied to drugs or animal tissues for transplants.

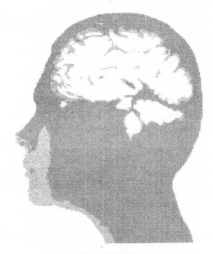

INDEX

Page numbers in **boldface** refer to a Figure or Table